T0223436

Scaphoid Fractures and Nonunions

Jeffrey Yao
Editor

Scaphoid Fractures and Nonunions

A Clinical Casebook

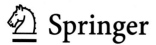 Springer

Editor
Jeffrey Yao, MD
Associate Professor of Orthopedic Surgery
Robert A. Chase Hand and Upper Limb Center,
Stanford University Medical Center
Palo Alto, CA, USA

ISBN 978-3-319-18976-5   ISBN 978-3-319-18977-2 (eBook)
DOI 10.1007/978-3-319-18977-2

Library of Congress Control Number: 2015943685

Springer Cham Heidelberg New York Dordrecht London

Printed on acid-free paper

Springer International Publishing AG Switzerland is part of Springer Science+
Business Media (www.springer.com)

Preface

The scaphoid is the most important bone in the wrist due to its involvement in multiple articulations. Fractures of the scaphoid, if neglected, will reliably lead to alterations in the biomechanics of the entire wrist. Dealing with these injuries remains an area of continuous discussion, debate, and discovery. It is with great pleasure that we present this work on the anatomy, diagnosis, and treatment of scaphoid fractures and nonunions.

The format of this casebook is slightly different than that of traditional textbooks. It is intended to be a quick reference guide for the indications and techniques (with clinical pearls) of all of the currently available methods of treating scaphoid fractures and nonunions. The concepts embodied within each of these chapters are presented in the form of a representative clinical case. How the patient developed symptoms, was diagnosed, treated, and ultimately recovered is all presented in the context of a specific manner of treating each presentation of these common injuries.

Our authors discuss all facets of the treatment of scaphoid fractures and nonunions that are the current state of the art. We start with a review of the relevant anatomy and the epidemiology behind these injuries. Next, we discuss the conservative treatment of acute fractures, and then the various approaches to treat acute fractures surgically, in adults as well as children. The following chapters discuss all of the various methods of management of scaphoid nonunions. Last, if the scaphoid is no longer salvageable or there is evidence of scaphoid nonunion advanced collapse (SNAC) arthrosis, the common salvage procedures that have been described are presented. We believe this resource will be an important addition to the armamentarium of house staff in training as well as seasoned attending surgeons.

I am eternally grateful to the authors of the following pages for giving their time and efforts to compile such thoughtful manuscripts. I have learned an immense amount from these cutting edge articles and I believe our readers will as well.

I would also like to thank my many mentors, colleagues, trainees, and patients for their involvement in my continuous drive to challenge myself to look for the best ways of treating patients with hand and upper extremity disorders.

Thank you to Margaret Burns and Kristopher Spring at Springer for their guidance throughout the process of conception, organization, development, and completion of this work. I would also like to thank Kanchan Kumari for her help as production editor and Dr Andre Cheah for his assistance in the final reviewing of the proofs.

Last, I would like to thank my wonderful wife, Jennifer. Without her continuous support and understanding, I would not be able to chase my academic pursuits. I could never overstate how much this is appreciated. I am also grateful for her unwavering, indomitable care of our two beautiful daughters, Madeline and Isabella, the most important people in my life who have given me the gift of life perspective and unmitigated joy.

Palo Alto, CA, USA   Jeffrey Yao, MD

Contents

The original version of Chapter 21 was revised. An erratum to this book can be found at https://doi.org/10.1007/978-3-319-18977-2_28

Contributors

Joshua M. Abzug, MD Department of Orthopaedics, University of Maryland, Timonium, MD, USA

Jared L. Burkett, MD Department of Orthopaedic Surgery and Rehabilitation, University of Mississippi Medical Center, Jackson, MS, USA

James Chang, MD Division of Plastic and Reconstructive Surgery, Department of Orthopaedics, Stanford School of Medicine, Redwood City, CA, USA

Harvey Chim, MD Department of Orthopaedics, Mayo Clnic, Rochester, MN, USA

Garet Comer, MD Robert A. Chase Hand and Upper Limb Center, Stanford University Medical Center, Palo Alto, CA, USA

Maurizio Corradi, MD Department of Orthopedic and Hand Surgery, Hospital University of Parma, Parma, Italy

Charles Day, MD, MBA Department of Orthopaedic Surgery, Beth Israel Deaconess Medical Center, Harvard Medical School, Boston, MA, USA

T. Del Gaudio, MD Clinic for Hand and Plastic Surgery, Orthopedic Clinic of Markgroeningen, Markgroeningen, Germany

David G. Dennison, MD Department of Orthopaedic Surgery, Mayo Clinic, Rochester, MN, USA

Roberto Diaz, MD Department of Orthopaedic Surgery, Stanford University, Redwood City, CA, USA

Christopher Doherty, MD, FRCSC The Roth|McFarlane Hand and Upper Limb Centre (HULC), Department of Surgery, Division of Orthopedic Surgery, University of Western Ontario, London, ON, Canada

Brandon P. Donnelly, MD Pontchartrain Orthopedics and Sports Medicine, Metairie, LA, USA

Olukemi Fajolu, MD Department of Orthopaedic Surgery, Beth Israel Deaconess Medical Center, Harvard Medical School, Boston, MA, USA

R. Glenn Gaston, MD Department of Hand Surgery, OrthoCarolina Hand Center, Charlotte, NC, USA

William B. Geissler, MD Division of Hand and Upper Extremity Surgery, Department of Orthopaedic Surgery and Rehabilitation, University of Mississippi Medical Center, Jackson, MS, USA

Mathilde Gras, MD Department of Hand Surgery, Institute de la Main, Clinique Jouvenet, Paris, France

Ruby Grewal, MD, MSc, FRCSC The Roth|McFarlane Hand and Upper Limb Centre, Department of Surgery, Division of Orthopedic Surgery, St Joseph's Health Center, London, ON, Canada

M. Haerle, MD Clinic for Hand and Plastic Surgery, Orthopedic Clinic of Markgroeningen, Markgroeningen, Germany

Warren C. Hammert, MD Department of Orthopaedics and Rehabilitation, University of Rochester Medical Center, Rochester, NY, USA

Thomas B. Hughes, MD Department of Orthopaedic Surgery, University of Pittsburgh School of Medicine, Pittsburgh, PA, USA

Jonathan Isaacs, MD Division of Hand Surgery, Department of Orthopaedic Surgery, Virginia Commonwealth University Health System, Richmond, VA, USA

Sidney M. Jacoby, MD Department of Orthopaedic Surgery, Thomas Jefferson University Hospital, Philadelphia, PA, USA

Sanjeev Kakar, MD, MRCS Department of Orthopaedic Surgery, Mayo Clinic, Rochester, MN, USA

Amy Kite, MD Division of Plastic Surgery, Department of General Surgery, Virginia Commonwealth University Health System, Richmond, VA, USA

Steve K. Lee, MD Department of Orthopaedic Surgery, Hospital for Special Surgery, Weill Medical College of Cornell University, New York, NY, USA

Peter R. Letourneau, MD Christine M. Kleinert Institute for Hand and Microsurgery, Louisville, KY, USA

Michael Lin, MD, PhD Alpine Orthopaedic Medical Group, Inc, Stockton, CA, USA

Robert C. Mason, MD Department of Orthopaedics and Rehabilitation, University of Rochester Medical Center, Rochester, NY, USA

Christophe Mathoulin, MD Institut de la Main, Hand department, Clinique Jouvenet, Paris, France

Nathan T. Morrell, MD University Orthopedics, Providence, RI, USA

A. Lee Osterman, MD The Philadelphia Hand Center, King of Prussia, PA, USA

James P. Higgins, MD Curtis National Hand Center, MedStar Union Memorial Hospital, Baltimore, MD, USA

Loukia K. Papatheodorou, MD, PhD Department of Orthopaedic Surgery, University of Pittsburgh, Pittsburgh, PA, USA

University of Pittsburgh Medical Center, Pittsburgh, PA, USA

Alessio Pedrazzini, MD Department of Orthopaedic Surgery and Traumatology, Oglio Po Hospital, Cremona, Italy

Peter C. Rhee, DO, MS Department of Orthopedic Surgery and Rehabilitation, San Antonio Military Medical Center, Fort Sam Houston, San Antonio, TX, USA

F. Edward Hebert School of Medicine, USUHS, Bethesda, MD, USA

Marco Rizzo, MD Department of Orthopedic Surgery, Mayo Clinic, Rochester, MN, USA

Tamara D. Rozental, MD Department of Orthopaedic Surgery, Beth Israel Deaconess Medical Center, Harvard Medical School, Boston, MA, USA

Alexander Y. Shin, MD Department of Orthopedic Surgery, Mayo Clinic, Rochester, MN, USA

David J. Slutsky, MD Department of Orthopedics, Harbor-UCLA Medical Center, Torrance, CA, USA

Dean G. Sotereanos, MD Department of Orthopaedic Surgery, University of Pittsburgh, Pittsburgh, PA, USA

University of Pittsburgh Medical Center, Pittsburgh, PA, USA

Justin D. Stull, BA Sidney Kimmel Medical College at Thomas Jefferson University, Philadelphia, PA, USA

Megan Tomaino, MPAS Department of Orthopaedic Surgery, University of Pittsburgh School of Medicine, Pittsburgh, PA, USA

Darrin J. Trask, MD Department of Orthopedics and Rehabilitation, University of Wisconsin School of Medicine and Public Health, Madison, WI, USA

Jonathan L. Tueting, MD Department of Orthopedics and Rehabilitation, University of Wisconsin School of Medicine and Public Health, Madison, WI, USA

Arnold-Peter C. Weiss, MD University Orthopedics, Providence, RI, USA

Department of Orthopaedics, Alpert Medical School of Brown University, Providence, RI, USA

Matthew Wilson, MD Carolinas Medical Center, Dept Orthopedic Surgery, Charlotte, NC, USA

Scott W. Wolfe, MD Hospital for Special Surgery, Weill Medical College of Cornell University, New York, NY, USA

Jeffrey Yao, MD Department of Orthopaedic Surgery, Robert A. Chase Hand and Upper Limb Center, Stanford University Medical Center, Palo Alto, CA, USA

Dan A. Zlotolow, MD Department of Orthopaedics, Temple University School of Medicine and Shriners Hospital for Children Philadelphia, Philadelphia, PA, USA

Chapter 1
Scaphoid Anatomy

Jonathan L. Tueting, Darrin J. Trask

The human scaphoid bone has a unique and complex shape that allows it to function as a critical element in proper wrist biomechanics. It is the only carpal bone that links the proximal and distal carpal rows. Its irregular anatomic shape and high percentage of coverage with articular cartilage lead to low tolerances during bony remodeling after injury. The scaphoid's ligamentous attachments, osseous anatomy, and complex biomechanics predispose this bone to certain ligamentous dysfunctions that lead to osteoarthritis, and certain fracture patterns that lead to malunion or nonunion. It also has a retrograde blood supply that leads to relatively high rates of avascular necrosis following fracture, particularly those closest to its most proximal end or pole. Injury to the scaphoid and its surrounding ligaments may significantly limit wrist function in the short term and can predispose patients to severe pain and osteoarthritis with concomitant long-term dysfunction.

J. L. Tueting (✉) · D. J. Trask
Department of Orthopedics and Rehabilitation, University of Wisconsin School of Medicine and Public Health, Madison, WI, USA
e-mail: Tueting@ortho.wisc.edu

© Springer International Publishing Switzerland 2015
J. Yao (ed.), *Scaphoid Fractures and Nonunions*,
DOI 10.1007/978-3-319-18977-2_1

1

Scaphoid Injury/Incidence

The scaphoid is the most commonly fractured carpal bone and accounts for nearly 70% of all carpal fractures [1, 2]. The most common injury mechanism is a fall onto an outstretched hand. Wolf and coauthors in 2009 studied 14,704 scaphoid fractures in a military population. They reported the unadjusted incidence of scaphoid fracture to be 121/100,000 person-years. Young males in the 20 to 24 year-old age group had the highest scaphoid fracture incidence at 164/100,000 person-years [2]. The same group studied the National Electronic Injury Surveillance System, which is a database of injuries presenting to emergency rooms in the USA. Over a 4-year period, 507 scaphoid fractures were identified in the database. When extrapolated, this corresponded to an estimated 21,481 scaphoid fractures nationally over the same time period with an estimated incidence of 1.47/100,000 person-years. They estimate that scaphoid fractures account for 2.4% of all wrist fractures, again with young males representing the highest risk for fracture [3].

Vascular Supply

The blood supply of the scaphoid predisposes it to avascular necrosis and nonunion following injury, particularly to the proximal pole. The radial artery provides the primary blood supply to the scaphoid [4]. In 1980, Gelbermann characterized the blood supply of the scaphoid by injecting latex into 15 cadaveric scaphoid bones. Approximately 70–80% of the intraosseous vascularity and the entire proximal pole are supplied from branches of the radial artery entering through the dorsal ridge [5] (Fig. 1.1). The large volume of bone dependent on a single intraosseous vessel poses a great risk to develop avascular necrosis following fracture [6]. Further studies showed that the scaphoid is the carpal bone at highest risk for avascular necrosis following injury [7]. The

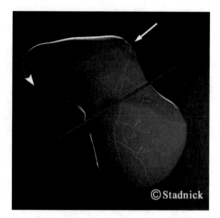

Fig. 1.1 Depiction of the typical blood supply to the scaphoid showing the larger distal dorsal branch supplying the proximal pole. (From http://rad-source.us/scaphoid-fracture/ with permission.)

remaining 20–30 % of the bone in the region of the distal tuberosity is supplied from volar radial artery branches [5] (Fig. 1.2). There is no apparent palmar-to-dorsal anastomosis. Venous drainage is via the dorsal ridge into the venae comitantes of the radial artery [7].

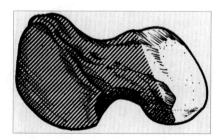

Fig. 1.2 Proximal 70–80 % of the scaphoid is supplied by the dorsal vessels (shaded) and the distal 20–30 % is supplied by the volar branches of the radial artery. (From ref. [5], with permission.)

Osseous Anatomy

The anatomy of the scaphoid presents a unique challenge when dealing with injury. Its anatomy has been described in detail by many authors [8]. The scaphoid is the only carpal bone to cross the proximal and distal rows and acts as a strut between them. It is the largest bone in the proximal carpal row, is oriented on an oblique long axis, and is concave volarly and ulnarly. Approximately 75% of the scaphoid is covered with articular cartilage, with only the volar surface being partially uncovered [9, 10]. Four distinct anatomic regions of the scaphoid have been described: (1) the tubercle, (2) the distal pole, (3) the proximal pole, and (4) the waist. (Fig. 1.3) In a study of 24 morphological and 11 morphometric scaphoid parameters, at least one morphometric feature was missing in 200 specimens. The scaphoid tubercle and dorsal sulcus were present consistently, with the greatest differences in waist circumference, size of the tubercle, and sulcus width [11]. A statistical model of scaphoid CT scans suggests that variations in morphology represent extremes of a normal distribution and not distinct subtypes [12]. The tubercle is directed radially and volarly and serves as an attachment point for the scaphotrapezoidal and the scaphotrapezial ligaments where it is also partially covered by the flexor carpi radialis tendon. At its distal end, the scaphoid articulates with both the trapezoid and the trapezium. However, a ridge along the scaphoid separating these articulations is not routinely identifiable [13]. At its proximal end, the scaphoid

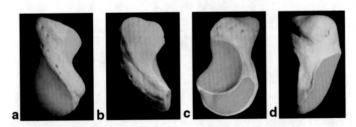

Fig. 1.3 Representative views of the scaphoid bone. Bottom of the image is proximal and the top of the image is distal. **a** Radial. **b** Dorsal. **c** Ulnar. **d** Volar. Colors represent articulations with other carpal bones: distal radius (green), trapezoid (orange), trapezium (yellow), capitate (blue), and lunate (red). (From ref. [8], with permission)

articulates with the scaphoid fossa of the distal radius. Along its ulnar border, the scaphoid articulates with the lunate proximally and the capitate distally [14].

Several studies have quantified the anthropometry of the human scaphoid. In 2007, Heinzelmann measured 30 cadaveric scaphoid bones with calipers. They found that male scaphoids were significantly longer than scaphoids in females (31.3 mm ± 2.1 vs. 27.3 mm ± 1.7). The male scaphoids were significantly wider than the female specimens when measured perpendicular to the long axis 2 mm from the proximal pole (4.5 mm ± 1.4 vs. 3.7 mm ± 0.5) and at the waist (13.6 mm ± 2.6 vs. 11.1 mm ± 1.2). This has significant implications in fracture fixation as diameters of many commercially available standard headless compression screws are close to the size of the proximal pole of female scaphoids. They suggest that the usual countersunk screw length will be 27 mm for males and 23 mm for females [15]. In a study that evaluated the scaphoid using three-dimensional computed tomography scans, Pichler showed that the scaphoid had a mean length of 26.0 mm and a mean volume of 3389.5 mm^3, again with a gender difference where length-adjusted female scaphoids are thinner [16]. Kivell showed that the female scaphoid body proximal-to-distal length is longer than that of males when size-adjusted; thus, as carpal size increases, female scaphoids are longer [17]. Lee characterized the osseous microstructure of the scaphoid. Articular regions showed the highest bone strength parameters (bone mineral density and trabecular density) and had thicker subchondral bone, especially at the articulations with the capitate and radius. The lowest number of trabeculae were found along the midcarpal side of the waist. Overall, the waist has thick subchondral and trabecular bone leading to a high moment of inertia against bending stresses[18].

Ligamentous Attachments

Numerous controversies exist within the literature regarding the ligamentous attachments to the scaphoid bone. The ligaments that attach to the scaphoid play an integral role in proper wrist biomechanics and function. A recent anatomic study by Jupiter analyzed eight cadaveric wrists with computed tomography and an imaging cryotome. Three-dimensional reconstruction showed ligamentous attachment consists of approximately 9% of total scaphoid surface area. The ligaments are divided into volar, dorsal, and scapholunate interosseous ligaments. The volar ligamentous complex connects the scaphoid to the distal radius and the adjacent of the carpal bones. The volar ligaments attaching to the scaphoid are made up of the radioscaphocapitate, scaphocapitate, scaphotrapezoidal, scaphotrapezial, transverse carpal, and radioscapholunate. The scaphocapitate ligament covers 40% of the volar ligament attachment surface area and covers nearly the entire ulnar scaphoid tubercle. Only one ligament attaches to the dorsal scaphoid; the dorsal intercarpal ligament originates from the dorsoradial aspect of the triquetrum and inserts on the proximal and waist areas of the dorsoradial ridge of the scaphoid. The scapholunate interosseous ligament is a single C-shaped ligament with a volar, dorsal, and proximal bundle dominated by the proximal portion of the ligament. These bundles are difficult to differentiate and can be viewed more as thickenings rather than discrete bundles [19] (Fig. 1.4).

All of these ligaments function to allow the scaphoid to serve a vital role in the complex biomechanics that are in play during normal wrist motion. Unfortunately, these interconnections also contribute to the abnormal and pathologic biomechanics that occur

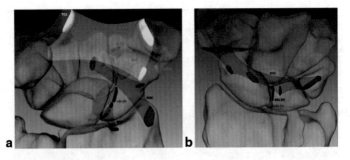

Fig. 1.4 Three-dimensional representation of the wrist showing the scaphoid ligaments and their attachments. Paths and attachments are based on cadaveric data. **a** Volar view. **b** Dorsal view. (From ref. [19], with permission.)

during injury to the scaphoid and/or its structural attachments. The following chapters of this text provide a detailed review of injuries to the scaphoid and the various treatment options that are currently available.

References

1. Sendher R, Ladd AL. The scaphoid. Orthop Clin N Am. 2013;44:107–20.
2. Wolf JM, Dawson L, Mountcastle SB et al. The incidence of scaphoid fracture in a military population. Injury. 2009;40:1316–9.
3. Van Tassel DC, Owens BD, Wolf JM. Incidence estimates and demographics of scaphoid fracture in the US population. J Hand Surg Am. 2010;35:1242–5.
4. Freedman DM, Botte MJ, Gelberman RH. Vascularity of the carpus. Clin Orthop Relat Res. 2001;383:47–59. Review. PubMed PMID:11210969.
5. Gelberman RH, Menon J. The vascularity of the scaphoid bone. J Hand Surg Am. 1980;5:508–13.
6. Gelberman RH, Gross MS. The vascularity of the wrist. Identification of arterial patterns at risk. Clin Orthop Relat Res. 1986;202:40–9. PubMed PMID:3514029.
7. Handley RC, Pooley J. The venous anatomy of the scaphoid. J Anat. 1991;178:115–8. PubMed PMID:1810919; PubMed Central PMCID:PMC1260539.
8. Buijze GA, Lozano-Calderon SA, Strackee SD, et al. Osseous and ligamentous scaphoid anatomy: part I. A systematic literature review highlighting controversies. J Hand Surg Am. 2011;36:1926–35.
9. Marai GE, Crisco JJ, Laidlaw DH. A kinematics-based method for generating cartilage maps and deformations in the multi-articulating wrist joint from CT images. Eng Med Biol Soc. 2006;1:2079–82.
10. Munk PL, Lee MJ, Logan PM, Connell DG, Janzen DL, Poon PY, Worsley DF, Coupland D. Scaphoid bone waist fractures, acute and chronic: imaging with different techniques. Am J Roentgenol. 1997;168:779–86.
11. Ceri N, Korman E, Gunal I, Tetik S. The morphological and morphometric features of the scaphoid. J Hand Surg Br. 2004;29(4):393–8. PubMed PMID:15234508.
12. van de Giessen M, Foumani M, Streekstra GJ, Strackee SD, Maas M, van Vliet LJ, Grimbergen KA, Vos FM. Statistical descriptions of scaphoid and lunate bone shapes. J Biomech. 2010;43(8):1463–9. doi:10.1016/j.jbiomech.2010.02.006. Epub 2010 Feb 24. PubMed PMID:20185138.
13. McLean JM, Bain GI, Watts AC, Mooney LT, Turner PC, Moss M. Imaging recognition of morphological variants at the midcarpal joint. J Hand Surg Am. 2009;34(6):1044–55. doi:10.1016/j.jhsa.2009.03.002. Epub 2009 June 4. PubMed PMID:19497684.

14. Berger RA. The anatomy of the scaphoid. Hand Clin. 2001;17(4):525–32. PubMed PMID:11775465.
15. Heinzelmann AD, Archer G, Bindra RR. Anthropometry of the human scaphoid. J Hand Surg Am. 2007;32(7):1005–8. PubMed PMID:17826553.
16. Pichler W, Windisch G, Schaffler G, Heidari N, Dorr K, Grechenig W. Computer-assisted 3-dimensional anthropometry of the scaphoid. Orthopedics. 2010;33(2):85–8. doi:10.3928/01477447-20100104-16. PubMed PMID:20192143.
17. Kivell TL, Guimont I, Wall CE. Sex-related shape dimorphism in the human radiocarpal and midcarpal joints. Anat Rec (Hoboken). 2013;296(1):19–30. doi:10.1002/ar.22609. Epub 2012 Nov 1. PubMed PMID:23125173.
18. Lee SB, Kim HJ, Chun JM, Lee CS, Kim SY, Kim PT, Jeon IH. Osseous microarchitecture of the scaphoid: cadaveric study of regional variations and clinical implications. Clin Anat. 2012;25(2):203–11. doi:10.1002/ca.21198. Epub 2011 May 5. PubMed PMID:21547958.
19. Buijze GA, Divinskikh, Strackee SD, et al. Osseous and ligamentous scaphoid anatomy: part II. Evaluation of ligament morphology using three-dimensional anatomical imaging. J Hand Surg Am. 2011;36:1936–43.

Chpter 2
Nonoperative Management of Non-displaced Acute Scaphoid Fracture

Megan Tomaino and Thomas B. Hughes

Case Presentation

The patient is a 15-year-old male with a history of left wrist pain following a football-related injury. He described the initial injury as hyperextension of his left wrist during football practice. He was seen at an urgent care center and initially diagnosed with a left wrist sprain. At that time, he was given a cock-up wrist splint. The patient continued to play football and "re-aggravated" his wrist 1 month later. He presented to a primary care sports medicine physician with left wrist pain. He reported that the pain had never resolved from a month earlier. New X-rays were obtained at that visit, an MRI was ordered, and the patient was removed from sports. The MRI was obtained about 1 week later and the patient was placed in a long arm cast and was referred to a hand surgeon for definitive care. He had no prior medical or surgical history, and he had no previous history of trauma to the left wrist. He denied tobacco use.

T. B. Hughes (✉) · M. Tomaino
Department of Orthopaedic Surgery, University of Pittsburgh
School of Medicine, Pittsburgh, PA, USA
e-mail: thughes424@aol.com

© Springer International Publishing Switzerland 2015   9
J. Yao (ed.), *Scaphoid Fractures and Nonunions,*
DOI 10.1007/978-3-319-18977-2_2

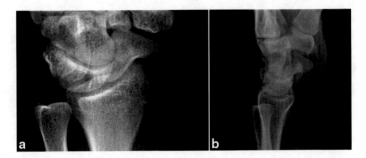

Fig. 2.1 An oblique radiograph **a** and lateral radiograph **b** obtained a day after the patient's injury. No true *AP* view was obtained. It is difficult to definitively identify a fracture line on these radiographs. (Published with kind permission of ©Megan Tomaino and Thomas B. Hughes, 2015. All rights reserved)

Physical Assessment

In the urgent care center on the day of the injury, the patient had point tenderness to the lateral side of the thumb, decreased grip strength, and mild wrist swelling at the radiocarpal joint. One month after the injury, the left wrist was mildly edematous with decreased wrist extension, focal tenderness in the anatomical snuff-box, and diminished grip strength of the left hand.

Diagnostic Studies

Radiographs of the left wrist on the day after the injury were interpreted as normal. These radiographs were subsequently reviewed by the upper extremity specialist and the scaphoid fracture could not be appreciated (Fig. 2.1). Repeat radiographs were obtained a month after the initial injury which are shown in Fig. 2.2. These demonstrated a minimally displaced scaphoid fracture. An MRI of the left wrist obtained 1 week later (5 weeks after the initial injury) revealed a non-displaced scaphoid waist fracture and intense

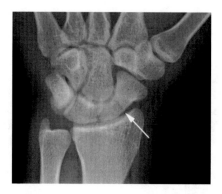

Fig. 2.2 An *AP* radiograph obtained 1 month after the injury clearly demonstrates an abnormality at the waist of the scaphoid (*arrow*). This, combined with persistent radial wrist pain, is enough to make the diagnosis. (Published with kind permission of ©Megan Tomaino and Thomas B. Hughes, 2015. All rights reserved)

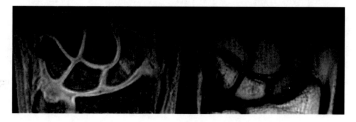

Fig. 2.3 Select coronal *MRI* demonstrating the fracture of the waist of the scaphoid. (Published with kind permission of ©Megan Tomaino and Thomas B. Hughes, 2015. All rights reserved)

edema of both the scaphoid and lunate. No fracture was identified in the lunate (Fig. 2.3).

Management Chosen

The patient was initially diagnosed with a left wrist strain and treated with a splint for 4 weeks. Initial recommendations for splinting and activities for the patient were nonspecific. It is clear that either the patient was noncompliant or the urgent care clinic was not explicit enough in their recommendations that the patient be immobilized, avoid wrist activities, and seek follow-up care.

When the non-displaced scaphoid fracture was suspected at 4 weeks, the patient was removed from sports, placed in a splint, and sent for an MRI. It was appropriate for the patient to be immobilized at this point (although some may recommend inclusion of the thumb in the splint, which was not done) and removed from football. It is unclear what specific advantage the MRI provided in diagnosis, treatment, or stratification of risks for this patient. After the non-displaced scaphoid waist fracture was discovered on MRI, he was immobilized in a cast for 7 weeks.

Clinical Course and Outcome

The cast was removed when there was radiographic evidence of scaphoid healing (11 weeks post-injury), and the patient had some wrist stiffness but no snuffbox tenderness. He was given a removable thumb spica splint and range of motion exercises for the wrist, but no formal physical therapy and he was not allowed to return to sport. The patient was encouraged to increase his activity as tolerated, but he continued to be restricted from participating in heavy lifting, football, or any sports. Fifteen weeks after the injury, X-rays demonstrated good healing of the fracture and the splint was recommended for comfort only. He was released to return to activities as tolerated, including football. At 15 weeks post-injury, X-rays revealed progressive healing of the mid-body fracture with good consolidation (Fig. 2.4). He had full range of motion of the left wrist, no pain, and he was able to return to normal activities.

Clinical Pearls/Pitfalls

- The key to identifying scaphoid fractures is to suspect them. The practitioner must be "aggressive" in the diagnosis of scaphoid fractures.

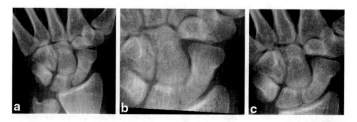

Fig. 2.4 *AP* radiographs obtained at 7 **a**, 11 **b**, and 15 **c** weeks after the injury demonstrate progressive healing of the fracture. (Published with kind permission of ©Megan Tomaino and Thomas B. Hughes, 2015. All rights reserved)

- Education of nonspecialists must continue as there is still a significant percentage of missed occult scaphoid fractures that have been seen by a practitioner that do not receive appropriate treatment or counseling. As more practice extenders are utilized in our health delivery system, this issue will continue to be significant.
- Patients with radial wrist pain need to be given specific instructions and limitations, including immobilization, in order to prevent scaphoid nonunions.
- Repeat imaging and close follow-up are critical for the successful treatment of the occult scaphoid fracture.
- When noncompliance is anticipated, advanced imaging may help establishing a diagnosis and lead to appropriate treatment.
- Complete bony union for scaphoid fractures takes several months. Even with occult fractures not visible on initial radiographs, healing can take three months or more.
- The results of nonoperative treatment are excellent with very few risks of complications. This approach to treatment should be considered for all non-displaced fractures and the risks of surgical intervention carefully weighed.

Literature Review and Discussion

The 15-year-old patient with a football injury in this case study represents a classic presentation of a scaphoid fracture. These fractures are most commonly seen in young adult males (age 15–40 years) after sports-related injuries or a fall on an outstretched hand. In recent decades, an increasing percentage of scaphoid fractures are occurring in young women, possibly because of increased participation in athletics [1, 2]. A typical description of the injury is a traumatic hyperextension of the wrist with radial deviation, such as described by the current patient during football practice. Patients often complain of generalized wrist or thumb pain and may not have pain over the scaphoid. Common physical exam findings include point tenderness over the anatomic snuffbox or thumb, decreased wrist range of motion, and weakened grip [1]. The current patient suffered from severe point tenderness over the thumb and weak grip of the left hand though radiographs interpreted as normal. The sensitivity of radiographs for scaphoid fractures can be as low as 70% and highly subject to the experience of the reader, resulting in easily missed fractures on initial testing [3]. Missed or untreated scaphoid fractures are at increased risk of nonunion, carpal collapse, and degenerative arthritis. Therefore, physicians should have a high degree of clinical suspicion for these injuries. In patients with vague symptoms about the radial wrist and thumb, the diagnosis must be excluded definitively prior to discharging the patient. Patients who are at risk for a scaphoid fracture should be placed in full-time immobilization, including the thumb, until the diagnosis is confirmed or eliminated.

Further testing with serial radiographs, a computed tomography (CT) or magnetic resonance imaging (MRI) scan is recommended. Serial radiographs may be effective. However, since several weeks of immobilization and activity modification are required between X-rays, there is a significant opportunity cost to this method of treatment. In order to return patients to sport and work faster, early advanced imaging can be helpful.

While CT scans are faster, widely available, and expensive, they are less reliable for identifying non-displaced scaphoid fractures.

CT scans do provide a better resolution of the anatomy of the fracture, in particular if the fracture is displaced and requires reduction. While some studies have shown CT scans to have poor sensitivity to displacement, it remains the best test available to assess displacement. In cases where initial radiographs are normal, it is very unlikely that displacement has occurred, and CT scans are probably unnecessary. However, in cases where there is an obvious fracture at initial presentation, CT scanning should be considered to assess displacement.

MRI is the most sensitive test to identify non-displaced fractures, and could have been helpful in this case had it been ordered after his initial evaluation at the urgent care clinic [1]. As it was not ordered until after the fracture was identified on the plain films, it did not aid in the diagnosis in this case. MRI can be useful to identify avascular necrosis, although this waist fracture was at limited risk for this problem [4].

Once the diagnosis of an acute non-displaced scaphoid fracture is confirmed, there are two main approaches to treatment: (1) nonsurgical immobilization and (2) surgical fixation. Both types of management ultimately aim to heal the fracture and avoid delayed union, nonunion, and avascular necrosis. Scaphoid fractures are at higher risk for these issues due to easily disrupted blood supply to the proximal pole. Branches from the radial artery supply the waist and distal tubercle; however, the proximal pole of the scaphoid relies exclusively on intraosseous blood flow, which can become disrupted with a fracture [1].

General considerations when evaluating the role of surgical and nonsurgical management include time to union, risk of nonunion, time to return to work or activities, functionality of the wrist, complications, overall cost, and patient satisfaction. Some studies have shown faster time to union, return to work, and return of range of motion with surgical fixation over casting, but others have found no evidence to support faster fracture union with surgical fixation [5–8]. In one randomized study, no statistically significant difference in time to union or rate of union was found in 53 patients with acute, non-displaced scaphoid waist fractures treated with either percutaneous screw fixation or immobilization for 10 weeks [8]. While patients managed nonoperatively cannot mobilize the wrist as quickly as surgical patients, the benefits of earlier mobilization after surgery may be transient. Follow-up from 12 months to 10 years after fracture has shown no statistically significant difference in fracture union, ROM, or patient satisfaction [7, 9–11].

Surgical treatment may be considered over immobilization in cases where the patient needs to return to work without a cast sooner. While it may seem that laborers are likely to gain the most from operative treatment, it may be those that do lighter tasks that can actually return to work sooner. Occupation is a significant factor in the consideration of surgery versus conservative treatment as self-employed and patients in nonmanual labor positions generally return to work faster than those in manual jobs, regardless of treatment [7, 12]. Surgical fixation may favored when the patient is employed in a job that is precluded by cast treatment because they are able to return to work sooner without a cast [8, 11, 13]. It should be noted that attitudes of the patient, employer, insurance company, and socioeconomic status of the patient are also significant factors in time to return to work [9, 12].

An additional consideration in developing treatment plans are complications. The literature has demonstrated a higher rate of complication with surgical treatment over conservative treatment [9, 14]. Short-term complications of surgery include prominent hardware, technical difficulties, infection, complex regional pain syndrome, and scar-related problems, whereas long-term complications include scaphotrapezial and scaphotrapeziotrapezoid joint osteoarthritis. The higher rate of arthritis with surgical treatment is thought to be from disruption of the scaphoid cartilage with screw fixation, although scaphotrapezial osteoarthritis is found in a small percentage of patients managed nonoperatively as well [10, 13, 15]. Additional complications noted in a small population of nonsurgical patients included intercalated segment instability discovered at 7-year follow-up. It has been suggested the instability in these cases may also be associated with a ligamentous injury at the time of fracture [11].

While there has been recent literature to support operative treatment of non-displaced fractures, there are certainly significant risks to surgical treatment that cannot be ignored. Based on these risks, some authors, such as Dias et al., developed an "aggressive conservative treatment" approach [9, 11]. Other authors have adopted a variation of this treatment approach which generally includes "aggressive" early diagnosis of the fracture and immobilizing all patients unless they have immediate cause for surgical fixation [15–17]. Early diagnosis and immobilization is important in preventing nonunion, and therefore, any patient suspected of having a scaphoid injury should be evaluated carefully with radiographs and possibly a CT or MRI.

The optimal cast for immobilizing an established scaphoid fracture has been studied; however, no significant differences in union rate have been noted with long arm, short arm, or thumb spica casts [17, 18]. A short arm thumb spica cast is generally accepted [14]; however, some institutions use a short arm cast with 20° wrist dorsiflexion and leaving the thumb free for scaphoid fractures [9, 11, 19]. A recent study has even demonstrated that in patients where the thumb is not included, there is a greater extent of healing compared to those in whom the thumb is immobilized [18]. The following algorithm compromises between both practices. If the scaphoid fracture is diagnosed via radiographs, and is non-displaced, a thumb spica cast should be applied initially. These fractures are less stable than more subtle injuries and fear of further displacement is warranted. At 6 weeks, if there is no displacement, or early signs of healing, it can be converted to a short arm cast without the inclusion of the thumb. If the initial radiographs are normal, and the diagnosis is made through serial radiographs or advanced imaging, this fracture is inherently stable and a short arm cast leaving the thumb free for 6–8 weeks can be applied. Regardless of the cast type, all patients should be re-evaluated with radiographs after 6–8 weeks. If radiographs show significant healing, a cast does not need to be reapplied. If radiographs do not clearly demonstrate healing at 6–8 weeks, a CT scan may be needed to assess healing at that point. Once 50% of the fracture has bridging bone, the patient can be given a removable splint for comfort and return to activities of daily living as tolerated. All patients should be re-evaluated with radiographs again to ensure fracture healing between 12 and 16 weeks postfracture. Patients with clear signs of nonunion, such as fracture motion and vacuolization, are recommended for surgical fixation.

In deciding to manage an acute non-displaced scaphoid fracture with an "aggressive conservative" treatment plan or surgical fixation, having a discussion with the patient regarding the potential risks and benefits of both surgical and nonsurgical treatment is essential. Besides the potential complications of surgery or immobilization, a significant concern for the patient is return to work and activity. These needs for return to activity must be carefully weighed against the higher risk of surgical complications seen with operative management. Both surgical and conservative treatment plans show no significant difference in union, rate of nonunion, or range of motion, and the conservative approach avoids the increased risk of complication associated with surgical fixation.

References

1. Kawamura K, Chung KC. Treatment of scaphoid fractures and nonunions. J Hand Surg. 2008;33A:988–97.
2. Van Tassel DC, Owens BD, Moriatis J. Incidence estimates and demographics of scaphoid fracture in the U.S. population. J Hand Surg. 2010;35A:1242–5.
3. Galer C, Kuka C, Breitenseher MJ, Trattnig S, Vecsei V. Diagnosis of occult scaphoid fractures and other wrist injuries. Are repeated clinical examinations and plain radiographs still state of the art? Langenbecks Arch Sug. 2001;120:73e–89e.
4. Lutsky K. Preoperative magnetic resonance imaging for evaluating scaphoid nonunion. J Hand Surg. 2012;37A;2383–5.
5. MCQueen MM, Gelbke MK, Wakefield A, Will EM, Gaebler C. Percutaneous screw fixation versus conservative treatment for fractures of the waist of the scaphoid. J Bone Jt Surg. 2008;90B:66–71.
6. Bond CD, Shin AY, McBride MT, Dao KD. Percutaneous screw fixation or cast immobilization for nondisplaced scaphoid fractures. J Bone Jt Surg. 2001;83A:4:483–88.
7. Buijze GA, Doornberg JN, Ham JS, Ring D, Bhandari M, Poolman RW. Surgical compared with conservative treatment acute nondisplaced or minimally displaced scaphoid fractures: a systemic review and meta-analysis of randomized controlled trials. J Bone Jt Surg Am. 2010;92:1534–44
8. Adolfson L, Lindau T, Arner M. Acutrak screw fixation versus cast immobilization for undisplaced scaphoid waist fractures. J Hand Surg. 2001;26B:3:192–5.

9. Dias JJ, Wildin CJ, Bhowal B, Thompson JR. Should acute scaphoid fractures be fixed? A randomized controlled trial. J Bone Jt Surg. 2005;87A:2160–8.

10. Vinnars B, Pietreaunu M, Bodestedt A, Ekenstam F, Gerdin B. Nonoperative compared with operative treatment of acute scaphoid fractures: a randomized clinical trial. J Bone Jt Surg. 2008;90:1176–85.

11. Dias JJ, Dhukaram V, Abhinav A, Bhowal B, Wildin CJ. Clinical and radiological outcome of cast immobilization versus surgical treatment of acute scaphoid fractures at a mean follow-up of 93 months. J Bone Jt Surg. 2008;90B:899–905.

12. Vinnars B, Ekenstam F, Gerdin B. Comparison of direct and indirect costs of internal fixation and cast treatment in acute scaphoid fractures: a randomized trial involving 52 patients. Acta Orthop. 2007;78:672–9.

13. Saeden B, Tornkvist H, Ponzer S, Hoglund M. Fracture of the carpal scaphoid: a prosepctive, randomised 12-year follow-up comparing operative and conservative treatment. J Bone Jt Surg. 2001;83B:230–4.

14. Ibrahim T, Qureshi A, Sutton AJ, Dias JJ. Minimally displaced and undisplaced scaphoid waist fractures: pairwise and network meta-analysis of randomized controlled trials. J Hand Surg. 2011;36-A:1759–68

15. Ibrahim T, Qureshi A, Sutton AJ, Dias J. Surgical versus nonsurgical treatment of acute minimally displaced and undisplaced scaphoid waist fractures: pairwise and network meta-analyses of randomized controlled trials. J Hand Surg. 2011;36A:1759–68.

16. Grewal R, King GJ. An evidence-based approach to the management of acute scaphoid fractures. J Hand Surg. 2009;34A:732–4.

17. Ram AN, Chung KC. Evidence-based management of acute nondisplaced scaphoid waist fractures. J Hand Surg. 2009;34A:735–38.

18. Doornberg JN, Buijze GA, Ham SJ, Ring D, Bhandari Mohit, Poolman R. Nonoperative treatment for acute scaphoid fractures: a systemic review and meta-analysis of randomized controlled trials. J Trauma. 2011;71(4):1073–81.

19. Buijze GA, Golings JC, Rhemrev SJ, Weening AA, Van Dijkman B, Doornberg JN, Ring D. Cast immobilization with and without immobilization of the thumb for nondisplaced and minimally displaced scaphoid waist fractures: a multicenter, randomized, controlled trial. J Hand Surg. 2014;39(4):621–7.M. Tomaino and T. B. Hughes

Chapter 3
Acute Scaphoid Fracture Management: Dorsal Approach

Robert C. Mason and Warren C. Hammert

Case Presentation

A 12-year-old right-hand dominant healthy male presented with right wrist pain that has persisted for the past 4 months after a fall onto his outstretched hand during a wrestling match. The patient was able to continue wrestling the remainder of the season. However, he had a noticeable wrist pain. Due to persistent discomfort in his wrist, his pediatrician evaluated him and radiographs were ordered (Fig. 3.1a, b), demonstrating a fracture. He was provided a referral for further care.

Physical Assessment

Physical assessment consists of history, examination, and imaging studies. A common mechanism for an acute fracture of the scaphoid is a fall on an extended and radially deviated wrist [1]. The history of the injury should be recorded, as well as immediate swelling, pain, and any previous injury, evaluation, or treatment. A

W. C. Hammert (✉) R. C. Mason
Department of Orthopaedics and Rehabilitation, University of Rochester Medical Center, 601 Elmwood Ave., Box 665, Rochester, NY 14642, USA
e-mail: Robert_mason@urmc.rochester.edu

© Springer International Publishing Switzerland 2015
J. Yao (ed.), *Scaphoid Fractures and Nonunions,*
DOI 10.1007/978-3-319-18977-2_3

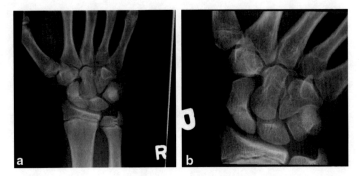

Fig. 3.1 a, b Pre-operative injury films—PA and Scaphoid view. (Published with kind permission of © Robert C. Mason and Warren C. Hammert, 2015. All Rights Reserved)

standard physical examination of the extremity should be completed, including evaluation of proximal and distal joints. Strength testing may be helpful in cases of delayed presentation but is of limited efficacy on the acute setting due to discomfort. Tenderness and swelling may be present in the anatomic snuffbox and/ or the scaphoid tubercle. Other provocative maneuvers, which are not specific for scaphoid fractures but often present, include discomfort with axial compression of the thumb, the scaphoid shift maneuver, and radial and ulnar deviation of the wrist with the forearm pronated [2]. Our patient described pain with gripping and activities, but not a rest. The pain did not preclude him from participating in activities. He had mild swelling along the radial wrist and discomfort with palpation in the snuffbox and direct pressure on the distal scaphoid. His wrist motion was slightly decreased in extension and radial deviation when compared to the opposite side. He had no discomfort or limitations of motion in the hand, forearm, or elbow.

Diagnostic Studies

Initial imaging consists of plain radiographs of the wrist, including posteroanterior (PA), lateral, semipronated oblique, and scaphoid view (PA with ulnar deviation) [3]. Using this technique, 84 % of scaphoid fractures can be identified, whereas 16 % could be missed, necessitating the follow-up radiographs [3]. Magnetic resonance imaging (MRI) scans have shown to be very sensitive in determining fractures of the scaphoid even in the acute setting. It has been shown that MRI in a suspected, radiographically occult fracture has a high sensitivity (100%) and a high specificity (95–100%) [4–6]. MRI can also provide the added benefit of identifying other injuries in the setting of wrist or hand pain, such as ligament injuries, other nondisplaced carpal or radius fractures, and, if contrast is administered, vascularity [3]. Standard MRI shows only 68% accuracy when assessing vascularity of the proximal pole; however, gadolinium enhancement improves this to 83% [7]. The role of computerized tomography (CT) scan is limited for acute scaphoid fractures and is dependent on the need for evaluation of displacement, comminution, or a humpback deformity to aid in surgical planning. CT scans can be used for evaluation if an MRI is contraindicated after initial negative or equivocal plain radiographs. CT scans can improve the reliability of detecting scaphoid fracture displacement but has only slightly greater accuracy of fracture identification (80%) than plain radiographs (70%) [8]. When a CT scan is obtained for evaluation of the scaphoid, it should be obtained in the plane of the scaphoid [9].

A useful algorithm for diagnosis of scaphoid fractures was described in Kawamura and Chung. When a nondisplaced fracture was identified on plain film, then a CT scan can be utilized if needed to determine the amount of fracture displacement. If there is high suspicion of a scaphoid fracture and plain films are negative or equivocal, then an MRI is performed to determine whether a scaphoid fracture is present or not and whether there are other sources of potential wrist pain [1].

Diagnosis

Fractures of the scaphoid can be classified according to the anatomic location and orientation of the fracture, as these are important determinants of treatment. These variables are important as the vascular supply to the scaphoid enters the dorsal ridge and the distal tubercle, with the proximal pole receiving all of its blood supply via retrograde flow [9]. Scaphoid fractures are often categorized into thirds: distal, middle, and proximal fractures with the majority of scaphoid fractures (approximately 75%) occurring at the waist and an additional 20% in the proximal third. The least common overall location is the distal third which is more common in children than adults [2]. Orientation of the fracture is described as transverse or oblique and may have implications with displacement and placement of a screw when internal fixation is used. This patient was diagnosed with a transverse fracture of the waist of the scaphoid.

Management Options

Nonoperative Treatment

When the fracture is nondisplaced in the waist or distal pole, it has been shown to have greater than 90% union rate with immobilization alone [10–12]. Controversy exists over the use of long-arm thumb spica splints/casts versus short-arm thumb spica splints/ casts. Till date, there have not been any studies to suggest one style cast is better [11, 13–15]. There is recent evidence suggesting there is no difference in union rates or time to union when including the thumb or leaving it free [16]. The fracture should be immobilized until healed, but there is not a consensus on how to determine healing. Many surgeons recommend CT scan to confirm healing when managing scaphoid fractures in a cast.

Operative Treatment

Any fracture with greater than 1 mm of displacement as well as nondisplaced proximal pole fractures should be treated surgically due to the higher incidence of nonunion and osteonecrosis caused by the tenuous blood supply in the proximal pole [17]. Operative treatment has also been recommended for active individuals such as laborers and athletes who cannot withstand the prolonged

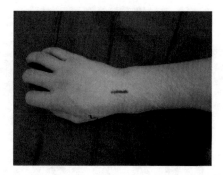

Fig. 3.2 Outline of dorsal incision. (Published with kind permission of © Robert C. Mason and Warren C. Hammert, 2015. All Rights Reserved)

immobilization. Internal fixation with a compression screw can reduce the period of immobilization and shorten the time to union [18]. The anatomical orientation of the scaphoid and the vascular supply lends the volar approach to the scaphoid as the path less likely to jeopardize the tenuous blood supply over a dorsal exposure [9]. A dorsal exposure is indicated for proximal pole fractures and nondisplaced to minimally displaced waist fractures with limited open or percutaneous fixation. The extent of the dorsal exposure will be determined based on the displacement and/or comminution of the fracture. If it is a nondisplaced fracture, a more limited exposure or percutaneous stabilization may be performed. Advantages of a dorsal approach are easier and more precise screw placement with central fixation. This is compared to the volar approach, which may lead to eccentric fixation and injury to the volar carpal ligaments and trapezium [1].

Dorsal Approach—Surgical Technique

The longitudinal incision is outlined from Lister's tubercle to the base of the third metacarpal (Fig. 3.2). The length of the incision may be extended in either direction if greater exposure is needed due to the displacement or comminution of the scaphoid fracture. The skin is incised and skin flaps are elevated off the extensor retinaculum proximally and at the level of the extensor tendons

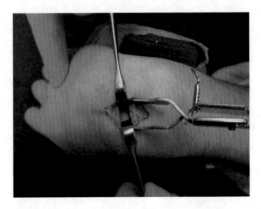

Fig. 3.3 Exposure of proximal pole of scaphoid. (Published with kind permission of © Robert C. Mason and Warren C. Hammert, 2015. All Rights Reserved)

over the wrist. The interval between the third and fourth compartments is identified, retracting the EPL in a radial direction and the EDC/EIP ulnarly. An oblique capsulotomy along the path of the dorsal radiocarpal ligament is made to expose the proximal scaphoid. The wrist is flexed and ulnarly deviated to expose the proximal aspect of the proximal pole (Fig. 3.3).

If greater exposure of the scaphoid is necessary for identification and reduction of the fracture line, a ligament splitting capsulotomy may be performed as described by Berger [19]. The posterior interosseous nerve (PIN) is sensory to the wrist capsule and runs along the radial aspect of the floor of the fourth compartment. Some surgeons advocate resecting a portion of this nerve to decrease pain from scarring of the nerve and resultant traction with wrist motion. The fracture is identified, and the alignment reduction is confirmed by visualization and fluoroscopy. For unstable fractures, a K-wire may be placed in the displaced fragment to aid in reduction by acting as a "joystick." After satisfactory reduction, the K-wire for the compression screw is placed 1–2 mm radial to the scapholunate ligament and it should be directed in a radial-volar trajectory toward the base of the thumb metacarpal. The wire should be placed along the central axis of the scaphoid, centrally in both dorsal/volar and radial/ulnar dimensions [20] (Fig. 3.4a, b). Fluoroscopy is performed with the wrist in flexion due to the entry point of the K-wire

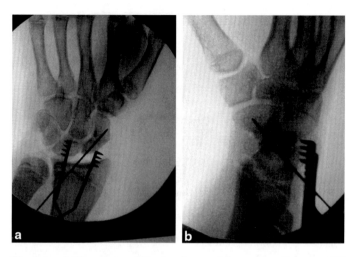

Fig. 3.4 a, b Fluoroscopy of K-wire placement for compression screw (*PA and lateral view*). (Published with kind permission of © Robert C. Mason and Warren C. Hammert, 2015. All Rights Reserved)

in the proximal pole. Alternatively, the K-wire may be advanced distally until the tip of the wire is deep to the articular surface and imaging completed and the wrist flexed and the wire advanced back proximally. Generally, a screw length 4 mm less than measured is chosen to allow for compression and burying the screw deep to the cartilaginous surface. After the length is determined, the K-wire should be advanced into the trapezium and a 2nd K-wire should be inserted into the scaphoid as an anti-rotational point to prevent displacement during screw insertion (Fig. 3.5). A cannulated drill is advanced to the desired length. When removing the drill, try to ensure the K-wire does not pull out with the drill. If it does, the wire may often be placed back in the tract and appropriate location should be confirmed with fluoroscopy. A headless compression screw may then be placed and should be countersunk deep to the articular cartilage. Fluoroscopy should be used to confirm reduction of the fracture and the appropriate position of the screw within the bone. The two K-wires are removed and the wrist is extended, and fluoroscopy is used to confirm fracture alignment and positioning of the screw.

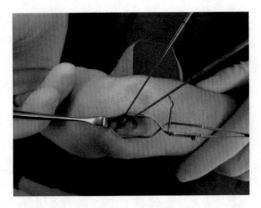

Fig. 3.5 K-wire placement (guide for compression screw and anti-rotation wire). (Published with kind permission of © Robert C. Mason and Warren C. Hammert, 2015. All Rights Reserved)

The capsule is closed, followed by the extensor retinaculum, if it was released, and the skin. We apply a short-arm thumb spica splint and obtain postoperative radiographs at 1 week. Proximal pole fractures or displaced fractures requiring reduction are immobilized for 4 weeks, and nondisplaced fractures are placed in a splint which is removed for hygienic purposes only at 1 week. Postoperative films are shown in Fig. 3.6a–d. Additional imaging is obtained at 4–6 week intervals until healing is confirmed [21].

Clinical Course and Outcome

At his final office visit, 3.5 months following surgery, he had no pain and symmetrical wrist and forearm motion with 60° extension, 65° flexion, 20° radial deviation, and 40° ulnar deviation. His forearm rotation was 85° supination and 80° pronation. Radiographs demonstrated normal carpal alignment with the cannulated compression screw in the scaphoid. The fracture line was no longer visible, consistent with radiographic healing. At this point, he returned to football and other contact activities without restrictions.

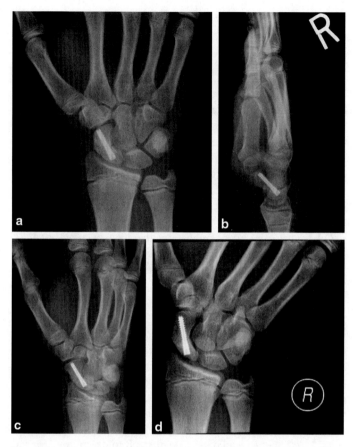

Fig. 3.6 a–d Postoperative films—PA, lateral, oblique, and scaphoid view. (Published with kind permission of © Robert C. Mason and Warren C. Hammert, 2015. All Rights Reserved)

Clinical Pearls/Pitfalls

- Proximal pole fractures require operative treatment due to the higher rate of nonunion and subsequent difficulty getting the nonunion to heal
- Other concerns with nonoperative treatment are frequent radiographs to check alignment, frequent office visits, stiffness with immobilized joints, and potential for skin breakdown [9].

- Surgery has associated risks, including injury to tendons and inappropriate screw placement with percutaneous approach [22].
- When performing fixation of small fragments and/or comminution, the fragment size will dictate the ability to use screws or the need for other means of fixation.
- For small proximal pole fragments, smaller screw size or headed, noncanulated screws may be necessary. In addition, temporary pinning of the scaphoid to capitate may be beneficial to limit motion of the scaphoid and allow healing.
- Even with optimal surgery, nonunion, mal-union, and failure of hardware can occur. Revision surgery is more complicated and may require additional bone grafting and prolonged immobilization.
- Other postoperative complications that have been reported are scar-related complications, prominent hardware, chronic regional pain syndrome, infection, and arthritis [23].

Literature Review and Discussion

A meta-analysis of 8 publications that provided data on 67 proximal scaphoid fractures managed nonoperatively reported a nonunion rate of 34 % [24]. Using this data, the relative risk for proximal pole fractures was calculated to be 7.5 in comparison with more distal fractures which have shown a union rate of ~90 % [10–12, 24]. Time to union can be difficult to determine. Grewal et al. used CT scans to predict union based on variables such as sclerosis, comminution, translation, and involvement of the proximal pole. Using this data, they were able to determine that time required to achieve union was significantly longer in proximal pole fractures in comparison with the waist and distal pole (113, 65 and 53 days respectively), with p-values in comparison with the proximal pole of 0.001 for waist fractures, and 0.008 for distal pole fractures. Within the same study, they found the presence of a humpback deformity and translation greater than 1 mm as significant ($p = 0.001$ and $p = 0.04$) predictors of nonunion [25]. There has been some suggestion of using CT scan to confirm final union prior to stating a fracture was healed due to the complex nature of the scaphoid [8, 26, 27].

Current opinion on displaced scaphoid fractures favors operative treatment due to the higher risk of malunion and/or nonunion [1]. Management of nondisplaced fractures is less clear. Bond et al. performed a randomized control trial involving 25 military personnel comparing percutaneous fixation to cast immobilization for treatment of nondisplaced scaphoid waist fractures. Time to union (7 versus 12—p =0.0003) and return to work (8 versus 15—p =0.0001) were significantly faster in the percutaneous fixation group [28]. This is comparable to other studies for the athletes or laborers that demonstrate an earlier return to athletic activities or work with internal fixation [18, 29, 30]. Cost analysis comparing operative and nonoperative treatment of nondisplaced scaphoid waist fractures suggests operative treatment is superior because it returns patients to work earlier [31, 32]. Davis et al. reported quality-adjusted life years (QALY) that operative fixation was more beneficial than casting. However, casting had a direct cost advantage over operative fixation [31]. Therefore, if a patient is dependent on hand function for income, surgery should be offered from a cost savings point of view. However, if they can accomplish tasks with a cast or their income is not tied to immediate recovery of hand function, then cast immobilization should be the treatment of choice [33].

References

1. Kawamura K, Chung KC. Treatment of scaphoid fractures and nonunions. J Hand Surg Am. 2008;33(6):998–7.
2. Haisman JM, Rohde RS, Weiland AJ. Acute fractures of the scaphoid: instructional course lecture. J Bone Joint Surg Am. 2006;88(12):2749–58.
3. Murthy NS. The role of magnetic resonance imaging in scaphoid fractures. J Hand Surg Am. 2013;38(10):2047–54.
4. Hunter JC, Escobedo EM, Wilson AJ, Hanel DP, Zink-Brody GC, Mann FA. MR imaging of clinically suspected scaphoid fractures. AJR Am J Roentgenol. 1997;168(5):1287–93.

5. Breitenseher MJ, Trattnig S, Gabler C, et al. MRI in radiologically occult scaphoid fractures. Initial experiences with 1.0 T vs 0.2 T. Radiologe. 1997;37(10):812–8.
6. Gaebler C, Kukla C, Breitenseher M, Trattnig S, Mittlboeck M, Vescei V. Magnetic resonance imaging of occult scaphoid fractures. J Trauma. 1996;41(1):73–76.
7. Cerezal L, Abascal F, Canga A, Garcia-Valtuille R, Bustamante M, del Pinal F. Usefulness of gadolinium enhanced MR imaging in teh evaluation of the vascularity of scaphoid nonunions. AJR Am J Roentgenol. 2000;174:141–9.
8. Lozano-Calderon S, Blazar P, Zurakowski D, Lee SG, Ring D. Diagnosis of scaphoid fracture displacement with radiography and computated tomography. J Bone Joint Surg Am. 2006;88(12):2696–702.
9. Ring D, Jupiter JB, Herndon JH. Acute fractures of the scaphoid. J Am Acad Orthop Surg. 2000;8(4):225–31.
10. Leslie IJ, Dickson RA. The fractured carpal scaphoid. Natural history and factors influencing outcome. J Bone Joint Surg Br. 1981;63:225–30.
11. Gellman H, Caputo RJ, Carter V, Aboulafia A, McKay M. Comparison of short and long thumb spica casts for non-displaced fractures of the carpal scaphoid. J Bone Joint Surg Am. 1989;71:354–7.
12. McLaughlin HL, Parkes JC 2nd. Fracture of the carpal navicular (scaphoid) bone: gradations in therapy based upon pathology. J Trauma. 1969;9:311–9.
13. McAdams TR, Spisak S, Beaulieu CF, Ladd AL. The effect of pronation and supination on the minimally displaced scaphoid fracture. Clin Orthop Relat Res. 2003;411:255–9.
14. Clay NR, Dias JJ, Costigan PS, Gregg PJ, Barton NJ. Need the thumb be immobilized in scaphoid fractures? A randomized prospective trial. J Bone Joint Surg Br. 1991;73:828–32.
15. Terkelsen CJ, Jepsen JM. Treatment of scaphoid fractures with a removable cast. Acta Orthop Scand. 1988;59:452–3.
16. Buijze GA, Goslings JC, Rhemrev SJ, et al. Cast immobilization with and without immobilization of the thumb for nondisplaced and Minimally displaced scaphoid waist fractures:a multicenter, randomized, controlled trial. J Hand Surg. 2014;39(4):621–7.
17. Russe O. Facture of the carpal navicular. Diagnosis, non-operative treatment, and operative treatment. J Bone Joint Surg Am. 1960;42:759–68.
18. Rettig AC, Kollias SC. Internal fixation of acute stable fractures in the athlete. Am J Sports Med. 1996;24:182–186.
19. Berger RA. Surgical technique: a method of defining palpable landmarks for the ligament-splitting dorsal wrist capsulotomy. J Hand Surg Am. 2007;32(8):1291–5.
20. McCallister WV, Knight J, Kaliappan R, Trumble TE. Central placement of the screw in simulated fractures of the scaphoid waist: a biomechanical study. J Bone Joint Surg Am. 2003;85(1):72–7.

21. Gholson JJ, Bae DS, Zurakowski D, Waters PM. Scaphoid fractures in children and adolescents: contemporary injury patterns and factors influencing time to union. J Bone Joint Surg Am. 2011;93:1210.
22. Adamany DC, Mikola EA, Fraser BJ. Percutaneous fixation of the scaphoid through a dorsal approach: an anatomic study. J Hand Surg Am. 2008;33(3):327–31.
23. Grewal R King GJ. An evidence based approach to the management of acute scaphoid fractures. J Hand Surg Am. 2009;34(4):732–4.
24. Eastley N, Singh H, Dias JJ, Taub N. Union rates after proximal scaphoid fractures; meta-analyses and review of available evidence. J Hand Surg Eur Vol. 2012;38(8):888–97.
25. Grewal R, Suh N, MacDermid JC. Use of computed tomopgraphy to predict union and time to union in acute scaphoid fractures treated nonoperatively. J Hand Surg Am. 2013;38(5):872–7.
26. Bain GI. Clinical utilization of computed tomography of the scaphoid. Hand Surg. 1999;4(1):3–9.
27. Temple CL, Ross DC, Bennett JD, Garvin GJ, King GJ, Faber KJ. Comparison of sagittal computed tomography and plain film radiography in a scaphoid fracture model. J Hand Surg Am. 2005;30(3):534–42.
28. Bond CD, Shin AY, McBride MT, Dao KD. Percutaneous screw fixation or cast immobilization for nondisplaced scaphoid fractures. J Bone Joint Surg Am. 2001;83-A(4):483–8.
29. Haddad FS, Goddard NJ. Acute percutaneous scaphoid fixation: a pilot study. J Bone Joint Surg Br. 1998;80:95–9.
30. Huene DR. Primary internal fixation of carpal navicular fractures in the athlete. Am J Sports Med. 1979;7:175–7.
31. Davis EN, Chung KC, Kotsis SV, Lau FH, Vijan S. A cost/utility analysis of open reduction and internal fixation versus cast immobilization for acute nondisplaced mid-waist scaphoid fractures. Plast Reconstr Surg. 2006;117:1223–35.
32. Papaloizos MY, Fusetti C, Christen T, Nagy L, Wasserfallen JB. Minimally invasive fixation versus conservative treatment of undisplaced scaphoid fractures: a cost-effectiveness study. J Hand Surg Am. 2004;29(2):116–9.
33. Ram AN, Chung KC. Evidence based medicine of acute nondisplaced scaphoid waist fractures. J Hand Surg Am. 2009;34(4):735–8.

Chapter 4
Acute Scaphoid Fractures: Volar Approach

Jonathan Isaacs and Amy Kite

Case Presentation

A 25-year-old right-hand-dominant male presented to our clinic complaining of left wrist pain after falling on an outstretched left arm 10 days earlier while playing basketball. An outside facility had diagnosed a scaphoid fracture and referred him for definitive treatment.

Physical Assessment

Moderate swelling was noted over the dorsal radial aspect of the left wrist. Point tenderness was noted at the anatomic snuffbox, and significant pain was noted with any wrist range of motion. The

J. Isaacs (✉)
Division of Hand Surgery, Department of Orthopaedic Surgery, Virginia
Commonwealth University Health System, Richmond, VA, USA
e-mail: jisaacs@mcvh-vcu.edu

A. Kite
Division of Plastic Surgery, Department of General Surgery, Virginia
Commonwealth University Health System, Richmond, VA, USA
e-mail: akite@mcvh-vcu.edu

© Springer International Publishing Switzerland 2015
J. Yao (ed.), *Scaphoid Fractures and Nonunions*,
DOI 10.1007/978-3-319-18977-2_4

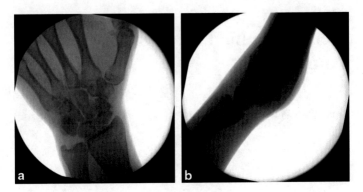

Fig. 4.1 Initial **a** PA, and **b** lateral radiographs demonstrating comminuted displaced scaphoid waist fracture. (Published with kind permission of ©Jonathan Isaacs and Amy Kite, 2015. All Rights Reserved)

patient's fingers were well perfused, and the patient had normal sensation to light touch.

Diagnostic Studies and Diagnosis

Initial fluoroscopy images of the left wrist revealed a comminuted and displaced scaphoid waist fracture (Fig. 4.1a, b).

Management Options/Management Chosen

Displaced scaphoid fractures have unacceptably high nonunion rates with nonoperative treatment, and surgical fixation is recommended. This patient was young, healthy, and active. There were no contraindications to undergoing surgery, and he was consented for elective open reduction internal fixation (ORIF).

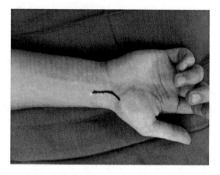

Fig. 4.2 Surgical incision for standard volar approach for scaphoid fixation. (Published with kind permission of ©Jonathan Isaacs and Amy Kite, 2015. All Rights Reserved)

Surgical Technique

Surgery was performed under regional anesthesia with tourniquet. A volar approach was chosen based on the location of the fracture as well as the humpback deformity. A hockey-stick incision was made over the distal flexor carpi radialis (FCR) tendon and angled radially and distally over the thenar eminence at the distal wrist flexion crease. Angling the incision in this direction avoids injury to the palmar sensory branch of the median nerve and exposes the scaphotrapezial joint for proper screw placement (Fig. 4.2). The FCR tendon was released and retracted in an ulnar direction to expose the volar capsule. The palmar branch of the radial artery was identified and efforts were made to protect it. The vessel occasionally needs to be tied off if preservation proves impossible. The scaphoid was palpated to direct the incision through the volar capsule and directly down onto the volar scaphoid tubercle. Starting distally and cutting proximally, we only released the tissue necessary to expose the fracture. Occasionally with this approach, we are able to preserve the important radioscaphocapitate ligament though in this case that was not possible. Still, we incised this ligament as cleanly as possible and maintained two stumps to facilitate later repair. The capsule was lifted off the distal pole of the scaphoid and the scaphotrapezoid joint opened to gain access to our screw "starting point." The soft tissues were released radially to expose the fracture though the dorsal radial blood supply was (and must always be) preserved. Wrist extension across a towel bump extends the scaphoid offering improved access to the volar scaphoid cortex. Hematoma and soft tissue were gently debrided from the fracture site using a combination of curettes, rongeurs, and bulb irrigation (applied under pressure). The fracture was assessed and preliminary reduction was attempted. The proximal pole and fracture line were stabilized by inserting a freer elevator around the radial aspect of the fracture and into the radioscaphoid articulation. Gentle volar–ulnar-directed pressure was applied to correct the extension deformity of the proximal pole (as it follows the lunate into an extended posture). The distal pole was reduced using a dental pick. Joystick Kirschner wires (K-wires) may be placed in the proximal and distal fragments if necessary to aid with reduction as well. Alignment was assessed along the radial and ulnar cortices of the scaphoid since the volar cortex in this case was comminuted. While maintaining the reduction, a guide pin was placed from the distal pole, down the scaphoid medullary canal across the fracture, and into the proximal pole. Because of the relative instability, we chose to place two (2.3 mm) screws and the guide pins were purposely placed to allow the insertion of two screws within the medullary canal. Alternatively, one guide pin can be placed down the center of the medullary canal for single-screw fixation. The guide pins were placed as dorsally as possible on the distal scaphoid at the scaphotrapezial articulation. The trapezium prevents this point from being too dorsal and, though it was not necessary in this case, the volar aspect of the trapezium may sometimes be rongeured off to facilitate pin placement. Sometimes several passes are necessary to place the pins into an acceptable position, but this is the essential step and poor screw placement will compromise scaphoid alignment and stability. Additionally, while repositioning a pin is relatively easy, gaining adequate purchase with a repositioned screw is challenging due to the limited amount of bone stock in the scaphoid.

Once pin placement and reduction were confirmed under direct vision as well as fluoroscopy imaging as acceptable, the appropriate screw length was obtained using the measuring guide. The

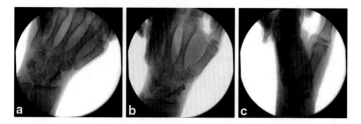

Fig. 4.3 Postoperative **a** PA, **b** oblique, and **c** lateral radiographs demonstrating reduced and anatomically aligned scaphoid fracture fixed with volar bone graft and two retrograde intramedullary screws. *PA* posterior-anterior. (Published with kind permission of ©Jonathan Isaacs and Amy Kite, 2015. All Rights Reserved)

guide pins were adjusted so that they were just abutting the inner cortex of the proximal scaphoid pole. 3–5 mm was subtracted from the measured length to account for cartilage thickness and compression at the fracture site (typically 2 mm for cartilage on either side and 1–2 mm for compression). The guide wires were overdrilled and cannulated screws placed one at a time though final tightening was performed by alternating between the two screws to ensure symmetrical compression. The guide pins were removed, and final live fluoroscopy imaging was used to evaluate screw placement, fracture reduction, and bone alignment (Fig. 4.3a–c).

The radioscaphocapitate ligament, followed by the volar capsule, was repaired using 3-0 braided polyester suture. The tourniquet was deflated and bipolar electrocautery was used for hemostasis before closing skin with 4-0 nylon sutures. A thumb spica splint was placed over a dry sterile dressing.

Clinical Course and Outcome

At two-week follow-up, the sutures were removed and a thumb spica cast was placed (due to degree of scaphoid comminution). At 6 weeks, the patient was advanced to a removable thumb spica splint and home range of motion exercises started. At 12 weeks, the patient demonstrated almost full range of motion without pain. The snuffbox was completely nontender, and fluoroscopy images demonstrated early healing. The patient was allowed to advance to activity as tolerated and elected not to return for further radiographic follow-up as he was deemed "clinically healed."

Clinical Pearls/Pitfalls

- Proper guide pin placement is essential to proper screw positioning and fracture stability.
- Pin, overdrill, and final screw placement can all go through trapezium (leaving a bony tunnel if necessary) to obtain desired position within the scaphoid.
- Ensure compression across fracture site as screw is tightened. If compression is not obtained:
    - Confirm that screw threads are across fracture line.
    - Reassess fracture reduction (especially rotational alignment).
    - Upsize the diameter of the screw to obtain better purchase.
- Roll the wrist back and forth under fluoroscopic imaging after fixation to evaluate for protruding screw threads and to confirm scaphoid alignment.

Literature Review and Discussion

The scaphoid is the most frequently fractured carpal bone, and while waist fractures account for 80%, fractures can occur at the proximal pole or scaphoid tubercle (distal pole) [1]. Falls onto an outstretched hand are the most common mechanism of isolated scaphoid fractures and occur typically in young men such as was the case in our patient [1–3]. As the scaphoid levers against the radius, the dorsal rim wedges into the scaphoid waist resulting in this characteristic fracture pattern [3].

Though this patient had obvious wrist trauma, symptoms of injury can be much less dramatic and scaphoid fractures are commonly missed. Swelling and radial-sided wrist pain as well as painful range of motion and point tenderness over the scaphoid tubercle or at the snuffbox following an appropriate mechanism of injury, all suggest the possibility of a scaphoid fracture.

Appropriate films including a neutral posteroanterior, oblique, lateral, and scaphoid projection views should pick up the majority of injuries though occult fractures do occur [4]. Temporary immobilization with repeat films in 7–10 days to allow early resorption at the fracture site may make the fracture line easier to see, though an MRI will also identify subtle scaphoid injury [2]. Missed scaphoid fractures are associated with high rates of nonunion [5].

Due to the unique anatomy, high biomechanical stresses, and an unfavorable local environment, scaphoid fractures are notoriously difficult to heal. With cartilage covering 75 % of the scaphoid surface and the scaphoid constantly bathed in joint fluid, bone healing can only occur by intramembranous ossification. That is, no stabilizing "callus" forms. Proximal pole extension forces transmitted through the ligamentous linkage to the lunate and distal pole flexion forces from normal axial loads across the wrist create a constant flexion deformity pulling the scaphoid into a "humpback" posture. Additionally, the tenuous blood supply due to limited arterial entry points at the dorsal ridge and distal third of the bone impedes healing and predisposes a relatively high risk for developing avascular necrosis. This risk is most notably for more proximal fractures but worrisome even with waist fractures [6]. Nondisplaced fractures in which inherent stability can resist these biomechanical deforming forces, allowing intramembranous healing and ingrowth of blood vessels, can be reliably treated with cast immobilization. Displaced or unstable proximal pole and waist fractures treated nonoperatively have high rates of nonunion [7].

The decision to repair this patient's scaphoid waist fracture was based on gross displacement and obvious instability though in many cases this is a much more difficult decision. Surgical indications, or clinical evidence of potential fracture instability, include any displacement greater than 1 mm, comminution at the fracture site, angulation through the fracture site, or displacement after a trial of nonoperative treatment. CT scans may be useful to better assess displacement or instability if plain radiographs are equivocal [6]. There are, of course, situations in which a patient's activity level precludes the prolonged immobilization necessary to achieve bony healing even with stable fractures, and many of these patients elect to undergo surgical fixation [8]. Proximal pole fractures have even longer nonoperative healing times and higher risks of avascular necrosis, and many authors now recommend initial surgical treatment of these regardless of stability [6]. Scaphoid tubercle fractures, on the other hand, typically heal rapidly with cast immobilization.

Scaphoid fixation can be performed either percutaneously or through an open volar or a dorsal approach. In this case, a volar approach allowed easy access to the fracture itself while protecting the already precarious blood supply [2, 3]. Additionally, the articulating proximal scaphoid surface was not violated as necessitated with dorsal screw placement. Dorsal approaches, however, offer better access for fixation of proximal pole fractures which are more difficult from a volar approach. The scapholunate ligament can be better assessed via a dorsal approach, and scarring of the volar wrist (with the volar approach) can result in loss of wrist extension [9].

Headless intramedullary compression screw fixation is the gold standard surgical fixation of scaphoid waist fractures. Though there are many different commercially available options, most achieve compression utilizing a thread differential between the two ends of the screw. In other words, the proximal screw advances more rapidly than the distal end resulting in a "relative" lag effect and compression across the fracture [5]. Multiple biomechanical studies have demonstrated some differences in screw stiffnesses but have failed to demonstrate definitive superior clinical advantage of one verses the others [10–13]. One of the most recent studies comparing compression of different screws shows four headless screws: Acutrak standard, Acutrak mini, Synthes

3.0, and Herbert Whipple, all having comparable compression [14]. Longer screws seem to control fracture motion more effectively [15], and while the biomechanical importance of central screw placement in the proximal pole has been demonstrated by McCallister et al. [16], fixation perpendicular to the fracture line may offer equivalent benefit in oblique fractures [17]. A second temporary parallel K-wire can resist rotation during screw placement with single-screw fixation for highly unstable fractures though this step, in our experience, is not necessary with stable interdigitation of fracture fragments. High union rates with volar reduction and retrograde screw fixation of acute scaphoid fractures have been reported in multiple studies [6, 18, 19].

We have started using double-screw fixation in large scaphoids and in situations of gross instability or bone loss such as demonstrated in this patient. Though definitive biomechanical studies of this construct are lacking, the principle that "wider" fixation achieves greater stiffness is well established [9]. Noting similar theoretical biomechanical advantages especially with torsional control, Garcia et al. recently reported the successful use of two-compression-screw fixation in the treatment of scaphoid nonunions [20].

Generic surgical complications can include infection, wound healing problems, and injury to neighboring vital structures. Articular injury from protruding screws due to malposition or inaccurate length can lead to arthritis [1]. Delayed unions and nonunions have been reported, and revision surgery can be considered in appropriate cases [6].

References

1. Meyer C, Chang J, Stern P, Osterman AL, Abzug JM. Complications of distal radial and scaphoid fracture treatment. J Bone Joint Surg Am. 2013;95(16):1517–26. doi:10.2106/JBJS.9516icl.
2. Adams JE, Steinmann SP. Acute scaphoid fractures. Hand Clin. 2010;26(1):97–103. doi:10.1016/j.hcl.2009.08.007.
3. Sendher R, Ladd AL. The scaphoid. Orthop Clin North Am. 2013;44(1): 107–20. doi:10.1016/j.ocl.2012.09.003.

4. Dorsay TA, Major NM, Helms CA. Cost-effectiveness of immediate MR imaging versus traditional follow-up for revealing radiographically occult scaphoid fractures. AJR Am J Roentgenol. 2001;177(6):1257–63. doi:10.2214/ajr.177.6.1771257.

5. Herbert TJ, Fisher WE. Management of the fractured scaphoid using a new bone screw. J Bone Joint Surg Br. 1984;66(1):114–23.

6. Kawamura K, Chung KC. Treatment of scaphoid fractures and nonunions. J Hand Surg Am. 2008;33(6):988–97. doi:10.1016/j.jhsa.2008.04.026.

7. Singh HP, Taub N, Dias JJ. Management of displaced fractures of the waist of the scaphoid: meta-analyses of comparative studies. Injury. 2012;43(6):933–9. doi:10.1016/j.injury.2012.02.012.

8. Ram AN, Chung KC. Evidence-based management of acute nondisplaced scaphoid waist fractures. J Hand Surg Am. 2009;34(4):735–8. doi:10.1016/j.jhsa.2008.12.028.

9. Haisman JM, Rohde RS, Weiland AJ. American academy of orthopaedic S. Acute fractures of the scaphoid. J Bone Joint Surg Am. 2006;88(12):2750–8.

10. Carter FM 2nd, Zimmerman MC, DiPaola DM, Mackessy RP, Parsons JR. Biomechanical comparison of fixation devices in experimental scaphoid osteotomies. J Hand Surg Am. 1991;16(5):907–12.

11. Newport ML, Williams CD, Bradley WD. Mechanical strength of scaphoid fixation. J Hand Surg Br. 1996;21(1):99–102.

12. Rankin G, Kuschner SH, Orlando C, McKellop H, Brien WW, Sherman RA. Biomechanical evaluation of a cannulated compressive screw for use in fractures of the scaphoid. J Hand Surg Am. 1991;16(6):1002–10.

13. Toby EB, Butler TE, McCormack TJ, Jayaraman G. A comparison of fixation screws for the scaphoid during application of cyclical bending loads. J Bone Joint Surg Am. 1997;79(8):1190–7.

14. Hart A, Harvey EJ, Lefebvre LP, Barthelat F, Rabiei R, Martineau PA. Insertion profiles of 4 headless compression screws. J Hand Surg Am. 2013;38(9):1728–34. doi:10.1016/j.jhsa.2013.04.027.

15. Dodds SD, Panjabi MM, Slade JF 3rd. Screw fixation of scaphoid fractures: a biomechanical assessment of screw length and screw augmentation. J Hand Surg Am. 2006;31(3):405–13. doi:10.1016/j.jhsa.2005.09.014.

16. McCallister WV, Knight J, Kaliappan R, Trumble TE. Central placement of the screw in simulated fractures of the scaphoid waist: a biomechanical study. J Bone Joint Surg Am. 2003;85-A(1):72–7.

17. Faucher GK, Golden ML 3rd, Sweeney KR, Hutton WC, Jarrett CD. Comparison of screw trajectory on stability of oblique scaphoid fractures: a mechanical study. J Hand Surg Am. 2014;39(3):430–5. doi:10.1016/j.jhsa.2013.12.015.

18. Rettig ME, Kozin SH, Cooney WP. Open reduction and internal fixation of acute displaced scaphoid waist fractures. J Hand Surg Am. 2001;26(2):271–6. doi:10.1053/jhsu.2001.21524.

19. Trumble TE, Gilbert M, Murray LW, Smith J, Rafijah G, McCallister WV. Displaced scaphoid fractures treated with open reduction and internal fixation with a cannulated screw. J Bone Joint Surg Am. 2000;82(5):633–41.
20. Garcia RM, Leversedge FJ, Aldridge JM, Richard MJ, Ruch DS. Scaphoid nonunions treated with 2 headless compression screws and bone grafting. J Hand Surg Am. 2014;39(7):1301–7 doi:10.1016/j.jhsa.2014.02.030.

Chapter 5
Arthroscopic-Assisted Management of Acute Scaphoid Fractures

William B. Geissler and Jared L. Burkett

Case Presentation

The patient was a 29-year-old male laborer status after a high-speed motor cycle injury. He presented to the emergency room with severe pain and swelling to his left wrist. He related that he was thrown off his motorcycle landing on his outstretched hyperextended wrist. Physical examination in the emergency room demonstrated a markedly deformed wrist with a moderate amount of swelling. He complained of paresthesias over the median nerve. Radiographs obtained in the emergency room revealed a displaced trans-scaphoid perilunate fracture dislocation of the left wrist (Fig. 5.1). At that point, under Bier block, a closed reduction was performed reducing the wrist.

The patient presented to the orthopedic clinic 1 week later with continued complaints of pain and swelling of the left wrist. There was less clinical deformity. He still had complaints of mild pares-

W. B. Geissler (✉)
Division of Hand and Upper Extremity Surgery, Department of Orthopaedic Surgery and Rehabilitation, University of Mississippi Medical Center, Jackson, MS, USA
e-mail: 3doghill@msn.com

J. L. Burkett
Department of Orthopaedic Surgery and Rehabilitation, University of Mississippi Medical Center, Jackson, MS, USA

© Springer International Publishing Switzerland 2015
J. Yao (ed.), *Scaphoid Fractures and Nonunions*,
DOI 10.1007/978-3-319-18977-2_5

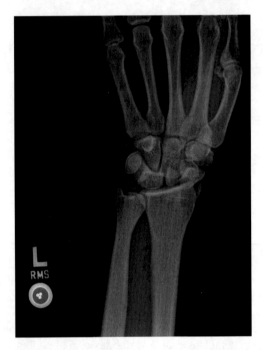

Fig. 5.1 Posterior Anterior (PA) radiograph of a trans-scaphoid perilunate dis-location. (Published with kind permission of © William B. Geissler and Jared L. Burkett, 2015. All rights reserved)

thesias over the median nerve which had significantly improved since the reduction.

Physical Assessment

Physical examination revealed moderate swelling of the wrist. He was point tender to palpation over the anatomic snuff box and the dorsal aspect of the scaphoid. He was also very point tender over the lunotriquetral (LT) interval. He had pain with a LT shuck maneuver. Sensation was grossly intact, including in the median nerve distribution. Digital range of motion was intact, but wrist range of motion was very limited due to pain.

Diagnostic Studies

Radiographs obtained in the clinic revealed the reduced trans-scaphoid perilunate dislocation. There was some widening of the LT interval, and the fracture line of the scaphoid was apparent on all views.

Diagnosis

Trans-scaphoid perilunate dislocation

Management Options

Traditional management would include open reduction and internal fixation of the scaphoid LT ligament repair and stabilization of the LT interval with Kirschner wires (K-wires) [1].The K-wires would be at risk for infection as they would be exiting the skin and would hamper rehabilitation. Other options besides open reduction were discussed including arthroscopic fixation of the fracture of the scaphoid and stabilization of the LT interval with a scapholunate intracarpal (SLIC) screw [2].

Management Chosen

Arthroscopic fixation of the scaphoid and percutaneous stabilization of the LT interval allows for earlier range of motion as compared to K-wire fixation and may also lead to decreased scarring for potentially increased range of motion. The SLIC screw (Acumed, Hillsboro, OR) is a screw that freely rotates at its midsection (Fig. 5.2). In addition, it has approximately 20° of toggle between the proximal and distal ends. When the screw is inserted, it allows a more normal rotation between the involved carpal bones. This allows the screw to be placed for a prolonged period of time,

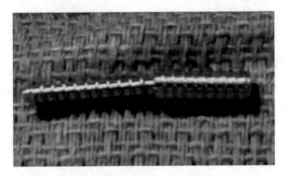

Fig. 5.2 View of the SLIC screw (Acumed, Hillsboro, OR). (Published with kind permission of © William B. Geissler and Jared L. Burkett, 2015. All rights reserved)

while the interosseous ligament heals allowing near-normal motion of the carpal bones with range of motion of the wrist. The screw can be taken out at approximately 6–9 months if the patient is symptomatic.

Surgical Technique

After general anesthesia is obtained, the patient is placed in supine position with the left arm outstretched on a hand table. A sterile tourniquet is applied at the level of the upper arm just proximal to the elbow crease. By placing the tourniquet more distal than normal at the level of the elbow crease allows better support of the upper extremity in the traction tower. The Acumed traction tower (Acumed, Hillsboro, OR) is set up on the hand table with the forearm plate in the dorsal position for easier removal later (Fig. 5.3). Traditionally, the forearm plate is placed on the volar aspect of the forearm for stability of the wrist which is slightly flexed in the traction tower. However, by placing the forearm plate dorsally, this allows for easier removal when the arm is flexed during the operative procedure. All bony prominences are well padded about the arm and forearm, and the skin does not touch the traction tower itself. The joint of the tower arm is set at the same level of the wrist joint, and the wrist is flexed approximately 30°. Finger traps are

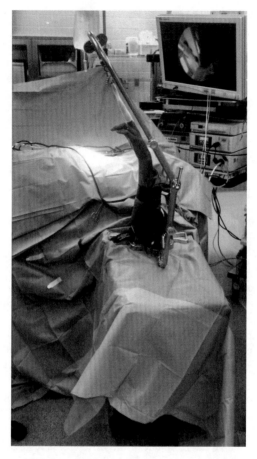

Fig. 5.3 Fluoroscopic view of placing the cannulated SLIC screw (Acumed, Hillsboro, OR) across the LT interval. (Published with kind permission of © William B. Geissler and Jared L. Burkett, 2015. All rights reserved)

placed along the index and long fingers, and the wrist is suspended with approximately 10–15 lb of traction. It is important that the bend of the tower is at the level of the wrist to allow wrist flexion in this procedure.

An 18-gauge needle is then initially placed in the 6U portal for inflow, and approximately 5–10 ccs of sterile lactated Ringers is injected into the radial carpal joint. An 18-gauge needle is then inserted into the radial carpal joint at the 3–4 portal (between the third and the fourth dorsal compartments) 1 cm distal to Lister's tubercle. It is important to place the needle at approximately 10° of angulation and volarly to match the volar tilt of the distal radius. The 3–4 portal is located down the radial border of the long meta-carpal. Once the ideal location of the 3–4 portal is identified, the skin is incised by pulling the skin against the tip of a no. 11 blade and blunt dissection is carried down with a hemostat to the level of the joint capsule. The 2.7-mm arthroscope with a blunt trocar is then introduced into the 3–4 portal.

Evaluation of this patient's radiocarpal space with the arthroscope in the 3–4 portal showed pristine articular cartilage to the scaphoid, lunate, and the distal radius. The scapholunate interosseous ligament was completely intact. Under direct visualization with the arthro-scope in the 3–4 portal, an 18-gauge needle is placed to localize the 6R portal. This enters the joint just distal to the articular disk of the triangular fibrocartilage complex. The arthroscope with a blunt tro-car is introduced into the 6R portal. Evaluation of the LT interval revealed a Geissler Grade IV tear of the LT interosseous ligament. Evaluation of the articular disk showed it to be intact with no tear.

The arthroscope was then introduced into the radial midcarpal space to evaluate the midcarpal joint. Evaluation of the radial mid-carpal space revealed the fracture at the waist of the scaphoid. It was displaced. Evaluation of the scapholunate interval with the arthro-scope in the midcarpal space showed it to be tight and congruent with no step-off. Continued evaluation of the ulnar side of the wrist again showed widening and separation of the LT interval consistent with a Geissler Grade IV injury of the LT interosseous ligament.

Carpal instability is best arthroscopically reduced by looking across the wrist to evaluate the rotation of the carpal bones. In this instance, the arthroscope was in the 3–4 portal. Joysticks were placed percutaneously into the lunate and triquetrum. Once the interval was anatomically reduced, a guide wire was placed in oscil-lation mode percutaneously through the triquetrum into the lunate. Using the oscillation mode helps protect the dorsal sensory branch of the ulnar nerve. The wrist tower is then flexed, confirming the ideal location of the guide wire in the LT interval with fluoroscopy. The guide wire is aimed toward the radial proximal corner of the

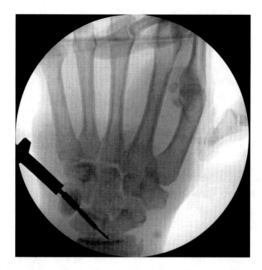

Fig. 5.4 In arthroscopic management of scaphoid fractures, it is best to set the forearm plate on the dorsal aspect of the forearm rather than the normal volar position with the arc traction tower (Acumed, Hillsboro, OR). In this manner, it makes it easier to flex the tower down to confirm position of the guide wire. (Published with kind permission of © William B. Geissler and Jared L. Burkett, 2015. All rights reserved)

lunate. Following confirmation of the ideal position of the guide wire, a 1-cm skin incision was made around it. A cannula with a blunt trocar is introduced to the level of the joint capsule to protect the dorsal sensory branch of the ulnar nerve. The SLIC cannulated drill was then placed over the guide wire and advanced between the triquetrum and the lunate, so the step of the drill is between the lunate and the triquetrum as confirmed under fluoroscopy. The length of the proximal portion of the screw was then measured directly by the drill under fluoroscopy. There are three optional lengths of the proximal portion of the screw. In this manner, the length of the portion is determined so that it will be flushed with the carpal bones to aid in its removal in the future. In this instance, a 25-mm SLIC screw was measured from the drill. This screw was inserted over the guide wire so that the interval of the screw would be exactly between the lunate and the triquetrum (Fig. 5.4). This will allow for near-normal carpal motion of the bones with range of motion of the wrist.

The traction tower was then placed back in the vertical position. The arthroscope was introduced into the radial midcarpal space to evaluate reduction to the LT interval. Evaluation of the LT interval with the arthroscope in the radial midcarpal space showed good stability and a congruent reduction between the lunate and the triquetrum.

The arthroscope was then transferred into the 6R portal and the scapholunate interval was identified. A probe was placed into the 3–4 portal to palpate the scapholunate interosseous ligament and the proximal pole of the scaphoid (Fig. 5.5). Following this, a 14-gauge needle is then introduced into the 3–4 portal into the radial carpal space. It is vital that the 14-gauge needle passes easily through the 3–4 portal without any resistance so as not to impale an extensor tendon. If there is any question, a hemostat can be used to spread the 3–4 portal and the needle placed over the hemostat

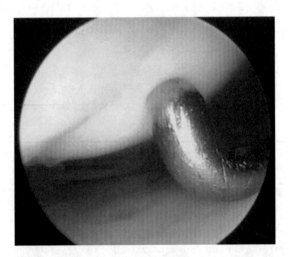

Fig. 5.5 Arthroscopic view with the arthroscope in the 6R portal. The junction of the scapholunate interosseous ligament and the proximal pole of the scaphoid is identified. This location is impaled with a 14-gauge needle. (Published with kind permission of © William B. Geissler and Jared L. Burkett, 2015. All rights reserved)

into the radial carpal space. The 14-gauge needle is then placed just radial to the scapholunate interosseous ligament into the proximal pole of the scaphoid. It is then impaled into the proximal pole under direct visualization with the arthroscope. In this manner, there is absolutely no guess work [3]–[4]. The exact location of the guide wire and eventually the position of the cannulated screw are directly visualized with the arthroscope under bright well-lit magnified conditions. Following placement of the guide wire, the arthroscope is placed in the midcarpal space to evaluate the reduction of the scaphoid fracture. Particularly, arthroscopy is very sensitive to detect malrotation of the fracture fragments as compared to fluoroscopy. A fracture of the waist is best seen with the arthroscope in the radial midcarpal space, and a fracture of the proximal pole is best seen with the arthroscope in the ulnar midcarpal space. If the fracture is not anatomically reduced as viewed with the arthroscope in the midcarpal space, the guide wire is advanced out distally from the proximal fragment while still being maintained in the distal scaphoid fracture fragment. Usually, manipulation of the tower and further extension and radial deviation will help anatomically reduce the scaphoid fracture. If this does not reduce it, the guide wire in the distal pole of the fragment can be used to manipulate and further reduce the fracture. Once the fracture is anatomically reduced, the guide wire is then advanced proximally into the proximal scaphoid fracture fragment.

The forearm strap is then removed along with the dorsally placed forearm plate, and the traction tower is flexed to be parallel to the floor (Fig. 5.6). The starting point at the most proximal pole of the scaphoid is then verified under fluoroscopy (Fig. 5.7). The ARC wrist traction tower is very fluoroscopy-friendly in that the traction bar is placed to the side of the forearm so as not to block the X-ray beam. Once the ideal starting point for the guide wire is confirmed under fluoroscopy, the needle is simply aimed toward the thumb. A guide wire for the mini Acutrak compression screw (Acumed, Hillsboro, OR) is then placed through the 14-gauge needle and aimed toward the thumb. Prior to advancing the guide wire under fluoroscopy, the appropriate trajectory and angulation of the guide wire is determined prior to its advancement into the scaphoid. The guide wire is then advanced under fluoroscopy to the far

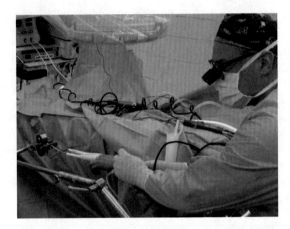

Fig. 5.6 The ARC traction tower (Acumed, Hillsboro, OR) is then flexed down to fluoroscopically confirm the ideal position of the needle. (Published with kind permission of © William B. Geissler and Jared L. Burkett, 2015. All rights reserved)

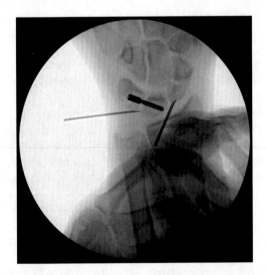

Fig. 5.7 Fluoroscopic view demonstrating precise placement of a 14-gauge needle on the proximal pole of the scaphoid. (Published with kind permission of © William B. Geissler and Jared L. Burkett, 2015. All rights reserved)

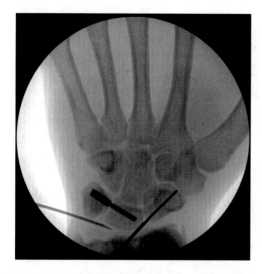

Fig. 5.8 Fluoroscopic view confirming placement of the guide wire down the central axis of the scaphoid. It is imperative to use a headless screw approximately 4 mm shorter than is measured. (Published with kind permission of © William B. Geissler and Jared L. Burkett, 2015. All rights reserved)

cortex of the distal pole of the scaphoid on the posteroanterior view under fluoroscopy. Ideal guide wire placement is then assessed on the posteroanterior oblique and lateral views under fluoroscopy to insure appropriate positioning of the guide wire down the center of the scaphoid (Fig. 5.8).This has been shown by McCallister et al. to be the optimum position biomechanically. The length of the screw is then determined by one of the two manners. Either the measuring guide is then used or an exact same length guide wire can be used. In this instance, a second guide wire was placed against the proximal pole of the scaphoid as viewed arthroscopically, and the difference in length between the two guide wires was measured. It is extremely important to use a screw at least 4 mm shorter than when using a headless compression screw [5–6]. A 24-mm headless compression screw was selected by measurement.

Prior to drilling and placing the screw, the guide wire is then advanced out the volar aspect of the hand and clamped with a hemostat to prevent pull of the wire during drilling as well as for easy retrieval in case the wire is broken during drilling and insertion.

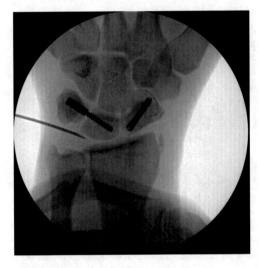

Fig. 5.9 Anteroposterior fluoroscopic view following stabilization of the trans-scaphoid perilunate dislocation. (Published with kind permission of © William B. Geissler and Jared L. Burkett, 2015. All rights reserved)

The scaphoid was then drilled through a soft tissue protector sleeve with the near-and-far reamers. A 24-mm Acumed mini Acu-trak screw was inserted over the guide wire leading to compression at the fracture site (Figs. 5.9 and 5.10). Following screw placement, the arm is brought back into the vertical position in the traction tower. It is very important to view screw placement with the arthroscope in the radial carpal space to insure that the screw is counter-sunk into the scaphoid and not protruding proximally.

Clinical Course and Outcome

Postoperatively, the patient was placed in a volar splint for approximately 2 weeks in 30° of extension with the thumb not included in the splint. Range of motion exercises were continued for 4 weeks.

Radiographs at 6 weeks postoperatively showed no loosening of the hardware. At that point, a range of motion and strengthening program through hand therapy was initiated. The patient was seen

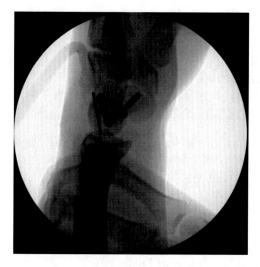

Fig. 5.10 Lateral fluoroscopic view confirming reduction of the trans-scaphoid perilunate dislocation. (Published with kind permission of © William B. Geissler and Jared L. Burkett, 2015. All rights reserved)

in approximately 3 months postoperatively. Range of motion of the wrist at that point showed 45° of extension, 30° of flexion, 10° of radial deviation, and 20° of ulnar deviation. The patient could make a full fist with good strength of 4/5. The patient clinically had no pain and was quite pleased. Radiographs showed bony consolidation of the scaphoid fracture and no loosening of the SLIC screw. The patient was then discharged to a home strengthening program.

Clinical Pearls/Pitfalls

- Clear arthroscopic visualization of the proximal pole of the scaphoid is mandatory. Any dorsal synovitis that may obscure visualization should be removed with a shaver.
- The starting point for the guide wire is the junction of the scapholunate interosseous ligament at the proximal pole of the scaphoid.

- Reduction of the scaphoid fracture should be visualized with the arthroscope in the midcarpal space.
- The position of the guide wire must be checked in posteroanterior, oblique, and lateral planes before reaming and insertion of the headless screw.
- A second guide wire may help to protect against rotation of the fracture fragments as the headless cannulated screw is being inserted.
- The position of the screw inserted in the scaphoid must be checked with the arthroscope in the radiocarpal space to ensure that it is not prominent.
- Final reduction of the scaphoid after screw insertion should be checked with the arthroscope in the midcarpal space.

Literature Review and Discussion

Haddad and Goddard reported their results in a pilot study of 15 patients with acute scaphoid fractures that were stabilized percutaneously through the volar approach [1]. Union was achieved in all patients in an average of 57 days, and range of motion at union was equal to that of the contralateral limb with their percutaneous technique. Grip strength averaged 90 % at 3 months.

Slade reported in a consecutive series of 27 fractures (17 waist fractures and 10 proximal pole fractures) treated with arthroscopic-assisted dorsal percutaneous approach [2, 3]. All patients underwent CT scans postoperatively which confirmed 100 % union rate in an average of 12 weeks. Of all the fractures, 18 of the fractures were treated within 1 month of injury.

Geissler reported on 13 patients with perilunate dislocations that were stabilized without K-wire fixation [4, 5]. Six of those patients had trans-scaphoid perilunate dislocations that were managed all arthroscopically. In the trans-scaphoid perilunate group, the arc of motion at 3 months was between 70 and 120°. Five patients had no pain. Stabilization of perilunate dislocations without Kirschner wires allows patients to participate in physical therapy at an earlier stage, resulting in a very functional range of motion at only 3 months postoperatively.

References

1. Haddad FS, Goddard NJ. Acute percutaneous scaphoid fixation using a cannulated screw. Chir Main. 1998;17(2):119–26.
2. Slade JF, Merrell GA, Geissler WB. Fixation of acute and selected non-union scaphoid fractures. In: Geissler WB, editor. Wrist arthroscopy. New York: Springer; 2005. pp 112–24.
3. Slade JF III, Grauer JN, Mahoney JD. Arthroscopic reduction and percutaneous fixation of scaphoid fractures with a novel dorsal technique. Orthop Clin North Am. 2000;30:247–61.
4. Geissler WB. Arthroscopic assisted fixation of fractures of the scaphoid. Atlas Hand Clin. 2003;8:37–56.
5. Geissler WB, Hammit MD. Arthroscopic aided fixation of scaphoid fractures. Hand Clin. 2001;17:575–88.

Suggested Readings

Kamineni S, Lavy CBD. Percutaneous fixation of scaphoid fractures: an anatomic study. J Hand Surg. 1999;24:85–8.
Whipple TL. The role of arthroscopy in the treatment of intraarticular wrist fractures. Hand Clin. 1995;11:13–8.

Chapter 6
Treatment of Acute Pediatric Scaphoid Waist Fractures

Peter R. Letourneau and Dan A. Zlotolow

Case Presentation

The patient was a 14-year-old right-hand dominant male who tripped on a tennis ball and landed on his outstretched left hand 1 week prior to presentation. He was evaluated by the emergency room and diagnosed with a scaphoid fracture. Initial treatment consisted of placing him in a removable thumb spica splint. He was then referred to a hand surgeon for additional evaluation and treatment. On presentation to the hand surgeon, he complained of mild-to-moderate intermittent pain. He denied any limitations in his activities of daily living. The patient was an elite tennis player and was eager to resume playing tennis as early as possible.

Peter R. Letourneau (✉) · Dan A. Zlotolow
Christine M. Kleinert Institute for Hand and Microsurgery,
Louisville, KY, USA

Dan A. Zlotolow
Department of Orthopaedics, Temple University School of Medicine
and Shriners Hospital for Children Philadelphia,
Philadelphia, PA, USA
e-mail: dzlotolow@yahoo.com

© Springer International Publishing Switzerland 2015
J. Yao (ed.), *Scaphoid Fractures and Nonunions*,
DOI 10.1007/978-3-319-18977-2_6

63

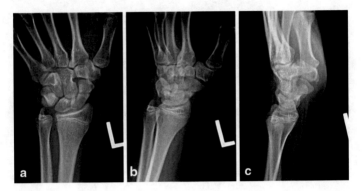

Fig. 6.1 Anteroposterior **a**, oblique **b**, and lateral **c** radiographs obtained shortly after the injury demonstrated a nondisplaced fracture of the scaphoid waist. (Published with kind permission of © Peter R. Letourneau and Dan A. Zlotolow, 2015. All rights reserved)

Physical Assessment

The physical examination was remarkable for mild ecchymosis and swelling over the dorsal radial left wrist and tenderness to palpation over the anatomic snuffbox. He also had diffuse ligamentous laxity, and both patellas were dislocatable.

Diagnostic Studies and Diagnosis

Left-wrist radiographs were significant for a nondisplaced scaphoid waist fracture and skeletal immaturity (Fig. 6.1). The scaphoid was completely ossified.

Management Options

Most acute scaphoid fractures that are minimally displaced or nondisplaced can be successfully treated with cast immobilization in the pediatric population. This patient was adamant about returning to full activity as quickly as possible; his coach was concerned that even a short-arm thumb spica cast would interfere with his ability to serve a tennis ball. Treatment options were reviewed with the family, including casting versus percutaneous screw fixation. The family was informed of the potential risks of percutaneous screw fixation, including injury to branches of the superficial radial nerve, infection, scaphotrapezial and radiocarpal screw prominence, nonunion, malunion, and fracture displacement during percutaneous fixation requiring open reduction and fixation.

Management Chosen

The patient chose to pursue percutaneous fixation because it would allow him the best chance to resume tennis more quickly.

Surgical Technique

Volar percutaneous screw fixation was performed using a modified technique to optimize screw position [1]. Ten pounds of traction was placed on the thumb, thereby facilitating reduction and opening the scaphotrapezial joint. Using a mini fluoroscopy unit to visualize the distal pole of the scaphoid, freehand K-wires were used to draw intersecting lines on the skin overlying the scaphotrapezial joint. A small incision was then made at the base of the thenar eminence over the scaphotrapezial joint, and a 14-gauge angiocatheter needle was placed into the distal pole of the scaphoid, starting within the scaphotrapezial joint. The angiocatheter needle facilitates localizing the starting point, directs the guide wire toward the proximal pole, functions as a lever to translate the trapezium ulnarly, and serves as a soft tissue protector. Proper placement was confirmed using fluoroscopy, and the needle was then gently tapped into position using a mallet. The guide wire was advanced across the fracture so that the wire ended up in the center of the proximal pole. Finally, the bone tunnel was hand-

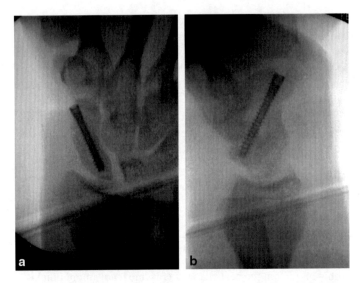

Fig. 6.2 Intraoperative fluoroscopic anteroposterior **a** and lateral **b** images show the percutaneously placed screw in place. (Published with kind permission of © Peter R. Letourneau and Dan A. Zlotolow, 2015. All rights reserved)

drilled, and a Mini-Acutrak 2 (Hillsboro, OR) screw was placed, making sure that the screw was at least 4 mm shorter than the measured length. Traction was released after the screw crossed the fracture site to allow for compression. Successful compression of the fracture was achieved. Final fluoroscopic images were obtained before the guide wires were removed and after the traction was released (Fig. 6.2). A sterile dressing and short-arm thumb spica splint were then placed.

Clinical Course and Outcome

Two weeks after the surgery, the patient was fitted with an over-the-counter thumb spica splint and he began some gentle range of motion exercises. Seven weeks after the surgery, routine X-rays demonstrated fracture healing and he was released to full activities without restrictions. At final follow-up 3 months postoperative, he had full range of motion in his left wrist that was equal to the contralateral side, as well as grip strength that was equal to the right. He denied any deficits in his activities of daily living and was able to resume playing tennis at his previous level of competitiveness.

Clinical Pearls/Pitfalls

- Failure to identify fracture on initial X-ray:
  Standard X-rays in children with incomplete ossification can be difficult to interpret; Initial X-rays should include the standard posterioanterior, lateral, and scaphoid views, and obtaining similar images of the contralateral wrist is useful. Failure to visualize a fracture in the context of positive physical examination findings does not exclude a fracture. These children should be immobilized in a short-arm thumb spica cast for 1–2 weeks and then reimaged. If clinical suspicion for a fracture persists in light of normal X-rays, obtaining an MRI may be appropriate, given that occult fractures can take up to 7 weeks to be seen on plain films [2, 3]

- Over-diagnosis of scapholunate dissociation:
  It is possible to over-diagnose injuries in the immature skeleton; the scapholunate interval appears abnormally wide until the carpal bones fully ossify, and failure to recognize this can lead to incorrect diagnosis of scapholunate dissociation ("pseudo-Terry Thomas sign") [4].

- Occult enchondroma:
  Occasionally, a patient will present with wrist pain without a clear mechanism of injury or history of only minor trauma; standard workup for a scaphoid fracture is still indicated given

case reports of scaphoid fractures as the initial presentation of occult scaphoid enchondromas [5].

- Combined distal radius and carpal bone fracture:

  The clinician must remember that clinical presentation of a scaphoid fracture can be subtle. It is critical to evaluate the wrist in the presence of more proximal injuries, keeping in mind that while distal radius fractures are much more common than scaphoid fractures, there are case reports of combined injuries [6].

- Bipartite scaphoid:

  There is some controversy regarding the possibility of a bipartite scaphoid. Some authors attribute this to a failure of fusion of the distal and proximal poles and regard this as a normal variant, while others argue that it represents a nonunion from a previous injury [7]. If seen on X-ray, the clinician should obtain images of the contralateral wrist as this rare variant, if it truly exists, would often be bilateral.

Literature Review and Discussion

This case illustrates one option for treating nondisplaced or minimally displaced scaphoid waist fractures in the adolescent. Scaphoid fractures are relatively rare in young children, but their incidence increases as children approach and enter adolescence. Overall, they represent 3 % of fractures of the hand and wrist, but only 0.45 % of pediatric upper extremity fractures, and 0.39 % of all pediatric fractures [7]. The low incidence of scaphoid fractures in younger children may be attributable to the cartilage cushion that protects the ossific nucleus. The ossific nucleus appears midway through the first decade of life and takes about 9 years to completely ossify [8]. As this cartilage cushion is progressively replaced by bone, the incidence of scaphoid fractures increases. The scaphoid ossifies from distal to proximal, and fracture patterns follow this ossification process with distal pole fractures being the most common scaphoid fracture in children 13 years and younger. However, a recent study of scaphoid fractures in children and adolescents found an anatomic distribution of fracture patterns that more closely resembles to those found in adults, with 71 % of fractures in the waist, 23 % at the distal pole, and 6 % at the proximal pole. Causes implicated in these recent epidemiological changes include the higher incidence of fractures in males, high-energy mechanisms of injury, closed physes, and higher body mass index [9].

The vast majority of pediatric scaphoid fractures will heal with cast immobilization for 2–3 months. Union rates for nondisplaced scaphoid fractures that are identified in the acute period approach 90 % [9]. This includes scaphoid tubercle fractures, waist, and proximal pole fractures. Indications for surgical intervention include fractures displaced greater than 1 mm or angulated greater than 10°, as well as chronic scaphoid nonunions [10].

With the increased participation in competitive sports in adolescence, seemingly more and more adolescent athletes and their parents' request return to full activity as soon as possible. In such cases, particularly when an early return to sports cannot be accommodated with a short-arm thumb spica cast, operative treatment may be offered and may minimize the time away from participation associated with the injury. However, surgical treatment does not necessarily guarantee a quicker return to full activity. For children with open physes, surgical fixation of acute fractures may not heal significantly faster than those treated with cast immobilization [9].

Since almost all acute nondisplaced scaphoid waist fractures will heal with cast immobilization, casting until radiological union is achieved is considered the standard of care for both the pediatric and adolescent patients. In addition, many scaphoid fractures in the immature skeleton will be distal pole fractures or monocortical fractures that are also suitable for casting

[7]. The case described here presents a patient who is reaching skeletal maturity and who is an elite athlete. Absolute indications for operative treatment in the skeletally immature patient include acute displaced waist and proximal pole fractures that are not likely to heal with cast immobilization alone [9].

Union rates using the described technique equal or exceed those treated nonoperatively [1]. Morbidity of the operative procedure is low, but complications can include technical errors that lead to scaphotrapezial joint arthritis, radiocarpal joint arthritis, injury to the superficial radial nerve, injury to the volar branch of the radial artery, infection, need to convert a percutaneous approach to an open approach, or exacerbation of an unstable fracture leading to compromise of the vasculature of the proximal pole of the scaphoid.

In conclusion, scaphoid fractures represent only a small proportion of fractures in the pediatric population. Vigilance is required since the implications of missing such an injury could be devastating, and include wrist arthritis and collapse (Fig. 6.3). It behooves all physicians, including pediatricians, emergency room physicians, and hand surgeons to have a high index of suspicion for occult fractures. The standard of care includes short-term cast immobilization if initial X-rays are negative, with repeat imaging in 2 weeks. If X-rays continue to be negative and there is still clinical suspicion for a scaphoid fracture, MRI may be indicated to confirm or deny the presence of a fracture [10]. Most acute scaphoid fractures that are minimally displaced or nondisplaced can be successfully treated with cast immobilization, but patient-specific factors must be considered when discussing individual treatment options.

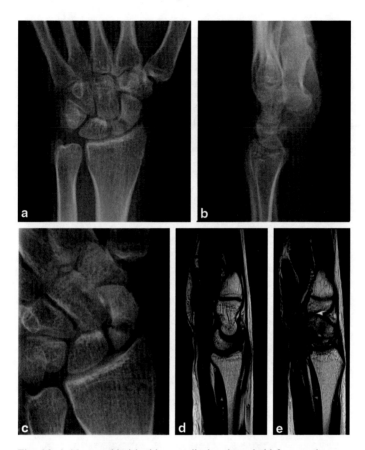

Fig. 6.3 A 15-year-old girl with a nondisplaced scaphoid fracture that was missed both by the emergency department and their radiologist, as well as the initial treating orthopaedic surgeon. She was treated in a removable splint for 2 weeks with no further follow-up. She presented to the same orthopaedist 4 months later with continued pain and now evidence of delayed union and a cavitary defect in the scaphoid on anteroposterior **a** and lateral **b** radiographs. She was again treated expectantly and returned 4 months later with an established nonunion on the scaphoid view **c** and a humpback deformity with Dorsal Intercalary Segment Instability (DISI) carpal instability on sagittal MRI **d**, **e**. (Published with kind permission of © Peter R. Letourneau and Dan A. Zlotolow, 2015. All rights reserved)

References

1. Zlotolow DA, Knutsen E, Yao J. Optimization of volar percutaneous screw fixation for scaphoid waist fractures using traction, positioning, imaging, and an angiocatheter guide. J Hand Surg. 2011;36(5):916–21.
2. Evenski AJ, Adamczyk MJ, Steiner RP, Morscher MA, Riley PM. Clinically suspected scaphoid fractures in children. J Pediatr Orthop. 2009;29(4):352–5.
3. Williams A, Lochner H. Pediatric hand and wrist injuries. Curr Rev Musculoskelet Med. 2013;6:18–25.
4. Light TR. Carpal injuries in children. Hand Clinics 2000;16(4):513–22.
5. Takka S, Poyraz A. Enchondroma of the scaphoid bone. Arch Ortho Trauma Surg. 2002;122:369–70.
6. Garcia-Mata S. Carpal scaphoid fracture nonunion in children. J Pediatr Orthop. 2002;22(4):448–51.
7. Christodoulou AG, Colton CL. Scaphoid fractures in children. J Pediatr Orthop. 1986;6(1):37–9.
8. Anz AW, Bushnell BD, Bynum, DK, Chloros GD, Wiesler ER. Pediatric scaphoid fractures. J Am Acad Orthop Surg. 2009;17(2):77–87.
9. Gholson JJ, Bae DS, Zurakowski D, Waters PM. Scaphoid fractures in children and adolescents: contemporary injury patterns and factors influencing time to union. J Bone Jt Surg (A). 2011;93(13):1210–9.
10. Huckstadt T, Klitscher D, Weltzien A, Müller LP, Rommens PM, Schier F. Pediatric fractures of the carpal scaphoid: a retrospective clinical and radiological study. J Pediatr Orthop. 2007;27(4):447–50.

Chapter 7
Scaphoid Nonunion: Surgical Fixation Without Bone Graft

Christopher Doherty and Ruby Grewal

Case Presentation

A 21-year-old right-hand dominant elite hockey player presented to our clinic with a known left scaphoid fracture. He sustained this injury 7 months ago while playing hockey. He was able to continue playing, albeit with wrist pain. He presented to the emergency room after the game and was diagnosed with a wrist sprain as no fractures were identified on initial radiographs. His pain gradually resolved over the course of 4 weeks and he returned to play the remaining 5 months of the season. He denies reinjuring the wrist, but noted a recurrence of symptoms when he started off-season training.

He complained of radial-sided wrist pain, exacerbated by activities causing loading of the wrist, particularly when bench press weightlifting. Another X-ray was performed, and an established scaphoid waist nonunion was identified. He was then immobilized

R. Grewal (✉)
The Roth|McFarlane Hand and Upper Limb Centre, Department of Surgery, Division of Orthopedic Surgery, St Joseph's Health Center, London, ON, Canada
e-mail: rgrewa@uwo.ca

C. Doherty
The Roth|McFarlane Hand and Upper Limb Centre (HULC), Department of Surgery, Division of Orthopedic Surgery, University of Western Ontario, London, ON, Canada

© Springer International Publishing Switzerland 2015 73
J. Yao (ed.), *Scaphoid Fractures and Nonunions*,
DOI 10.1007/978-3-319-18977-2_7

in a short-arm thumb spica cast and referred to our hand and upper limb center.

Physical Assessment

The wrist appeared normal, with no swelling or deformity noted on examination. He had pain with palpation in the anatomic snuffbox. He had normal range of motion of the digits and elbow. Flexion and extension of the affected wrist were 49° and 37°, respectively, compared to 79° and 59° on the unaffected side. The distal radioulnar joint was stable. Pronation and supination of the affected wrist were 80° and 82°, respectively, compared to 77° and 83° on the unaffected wrist. The hand had normal sensation within all nerve distributions. The Watson-shift test was negative, and the remainder of the hand and wrist examination was within normal limits.

Diagnostic Studies

Scaphoid X-ray views of the left wrist demonstrated evidence of a nonunited scaphoid waist fracture (Fig. 7.1a, b, c). Minimal sclerotic changes were evident adjacent to the fracture site. There were mild cystic changes and no humpback deformity. There was no evidence of a dorsal intercalated segmental instability (DISI) deformity or degenerative changes (i.e., scaphoid non-union advanced collapse (SNAC) wrist). A CT scan was performed to better delineate the fracture [1, 2]. CT was used because it more reliably identifies fracture displacement and angulation, especially when used in conjunction with X-ray imaging [1, 2]. Figure 7.2a and b is representative coronal and sagittal cuts of the scaphoid. The CT scan demonstrated mild cystic changes adjacent to the fracture, confirming that there was minimal sclerosis along the fracture line and no underlying humpback deformity

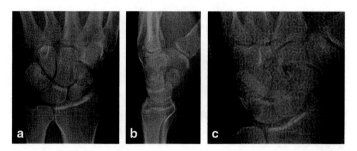

Fig. 7.1 Scaphoid views of the left wrist. **a** PA view demonstrating cystic changes at fracture site. **b** Lateral view demonstrating maintenance of normal alignment, with no humpback or angular deformity. **c** Oblique view featuring minimal displacement of the fracture. (Published with kind permission of © Christopher Doherty and Ruby Grewal, 2015. All rights reserved)

or displacement. An MRI was performed to rule out avascular necrosis of the proximal pole [3]. Figure 7.3 is a coronal cut of a T1-weighted MRI demonstrating scaphoid nonunion with no evidence of avascular necrosis of the proximal pole of the scaphoid.

Diagnosis

This patient was diagnosed with a scaphoid nonunion. As with many nonunions, it most likely occurred as a result of a missed scaphoid fracture, which we suspect occurred as a result of his injury 7 months ago. The chronicity of his injury (> 6 months) allowed us to classify it as a nonunion rather than a delayed union [4].

Radiographic findings (X-ray and CT) that supported this diagnosis included evidence of a fracture at the waist of the scaphoid without evidence of callus formation or bone bridging the fracture gap, mild sclerosis, and cystic formation [5]. Avascular necrosis (AVN) was ruled out based on the MRI.

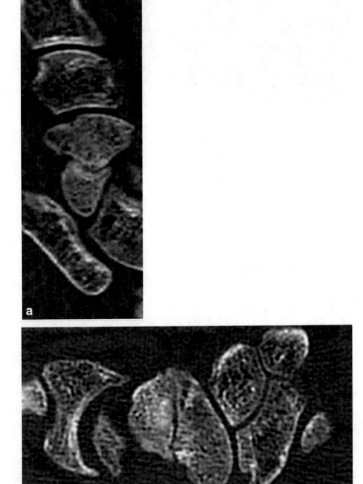

Fig. 7.2 Computed tomography of the left scaphoid. **a** Coronal cut demonstrating minimal sclerosis and mild cystic changes. **b** Sagittal view showing no humpback deformity and alignment of the fracture fragments. (Published with kind permission of © Christopher Doherty and Ruby Grewal, 2015. All rights reserved)

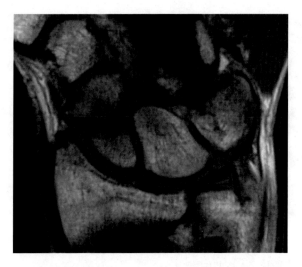

Fig. 7.3   T1-weighted MRI demonstrating scaphoid nonunion with no evidence of avascular necrosis of the proximal pole of the scaphoid. (Published with kind permission of © Christopher Doherty and Ruby Grewal, 2015. All rights reserved)

Management Options

The treatment goals for scaphoid nonunions are to achieve bony healing, correct any underlying carpal deformities, and prevent future arthritis. While it may be reasonable to offer a trial of immobilization in cases of delayed union, once patients are greater than 6 months from the initial injury, operative intervention provides a more predictable outcome. Surgical options for scaphoid nonunions include internal fixation (using an open, percutaneous, or arthroscopic approach) with or without bone grafting. The decision to perform internal fixation without the use of bone graft cannot be definitively made until the nonunion has been adequately evaluated. Evaluation includes careful assessment of the preoperative imaging and direct assessment of the scaphoid intraoperatively. Preoperatively, radiographic features that may suggest that a bone graft is not necessary include minimal sclerosis at the nonunion site (less than 1 mm), minimal cyst forma-

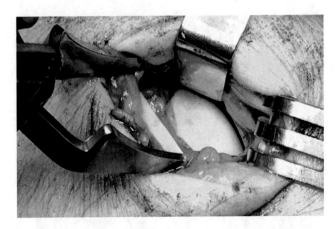

Fig. 7.4 Intraoperative evaluation demonstrating an intact cartilaginous cap. (Published with kind permission of © Christopher Doherty and Ruby Grewal, 2015. All rights reserved)

tion, no collapse or change in the architecture of the scaphoid, and normal vascularity of the proximal fragment [6]. If these criteria are not met, bone grafting will likely be required. The intraoperative evaluation of the scaphoid nonunion is a critical step, which helps to confirm whether bone grafting is required, as preoperative imaging may not always correlate with intraoperative findings [7]. Intraoperative evaluation of the nonunion can be performed open or arthroscopically [7, 8]. Intraoperative features that are compatible with fixation without bone grafting include an intact cartilaginous cap, evidence of only a faint nonunion fracture line in the waist of the scaphoid, no humpback deformity, minimal differential movement between proximal and distal fragments, and minimal sclerosis or resorption at the edges of each fracture fragment [8]. For example, Fig. 7.4a and b demonstrates an intact cartilaginous cap upon intraoperative inspection with radiographic evidence of a fracture in the waist of the scaphoid. Internal fixation without bone graft is generally reserved for non-to-minimally displaced fractures, within approximately 6 months of injury, that fit the abovementioned criteria [7–9]. Fixation should be rigid and in our experience this is best achieved with a headless compression screw, following the same technique as with an acute scaphoid fracture. Other methods of fixation (i.e., K-wire fixation) are not recommended as compression at the nonunion site is a key component of the fixation. Postoperatively, a variety of immobilization protocols may be used [6, 8]. If adequate rigid fixation is achieved, early active range of motion may be considered (2 weeks postoperatively) [8]. Alternatively, immobilization from 6 to 12 weeks may be used with an above or below elbow cast (thumb spica or Colles' cast) [6]. It is our preference to immobilize for 6 weeks in a short-arm thumb spica cast and then begin gradual range of motion exercises once union has been achieved.

Management Chosen

In this case, both clinical and radiographic factors contributed to our management decision. We did not entertain a course of further immobilization for two main reasons. First, the patient is an elite hockey player and wished to return to training as soon as possible. Second, a 6-week trial of cast immobilization had already been attempted with no further evidence of progression of union. Radiographic factors (based on preoperative imaging) and our intraoperative assessment contributed to our decision to perform internal fixation with a headless compression screw without bone graft. Based on preoperative imaging (Figs. 7.1 and 7.2), there was minimal displacement, no humpback deformity, minimal sclerosis (less than 1 mm), and no avascular necrosis. Given these factors, our level of suspicion for requiring bone graft was low. However, there was mild cystic formation on the imaging, and the duration since injury was 7 months; therefore, we felt inclined to visually inspect the nonunion intraoperatively. Intraoperative evaluation can be performed arthroscopically or via a volar open approach to the scaphoid. We generally use our preoperative level of suspicion for requiring bone graft to determine whether we assess the scaphoid arthroscopically or through an open volar approach. Arthroscopic evaluation provides the benefit of reduced morbidity if an open approach is not required for a bone graft; however, an open approach allows the surgeon to apply stress across the nonunion that may be more difficult to do arthroscopically. As described above, the duration since injury in this patient is beyond the 6-month window some authors describe for suitability of not requiring a bone graft [9]. Also, there was mild cystic formation at the nonunion site, so we therefore elected to do an open volar approach to the scaphoid because we felt that bone grafting may be necessary and prepared the patient for this possibility.

Surgical Technique

Intraoperatively, the location of the nonunion site was confirmed with X-ray. In this case, the fracture line was evident; however, the cartilaginous cap was preserved despite the presence of nonunion. The two fragments did not move differentially to one another. Therefore, the use of bone graft was judged not to be necessary. Next, the scaphoid was prepared for placement of an Acutrak 2 (Acumed, Oregon, USA) compression screw from distal to proximal. The screw was delivered and confirmed to be in adequate position using intraoperative imaging (Fig. 7.5a and b).

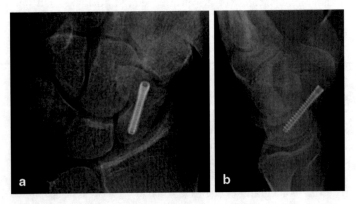

Fig. 7.5 Postoperative (2 weeks). **a** PA X-ray of the left wrist demonstrating hardware in good position with compression of the nonunion **b** and lateral X-ray of the left wrist with normal alignment of the scaphoid and no DISI deformity. (Published with kind permission of © Christopher Doherty and Ruby Grewal, 2015. All rights reserved)

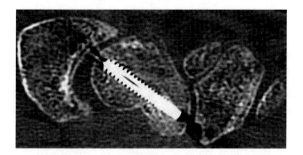

Fig. 7.6 Computed tomography at 6 weeks postoperatively showing evidence of union across the fracture with cannulated screw in good position. (Published with kind permission of © Christopher Doherty and Ruby Grewal, 2015. All rights reserved)

The patient was then placed in a short-arm thumb spica cast for 6 weeks. The patient was discharged home the day of the procedure. His postoperative recovery was unremarkable.

Clinical Course and Outcome

At 6 weeks postoperatively, the patient returned to the clinic and had a CT of the scaphoid to evaluate bone healing (Fig. 7.6). CT is chosen to evaluate union as opposed to X-ray because it is a more reliable modality, the cost difference is marginal at our center, and it provides a more definitive assessment of union [2, 10]. The cast was removed, and on physical examination, there was no tenderness to palpation over the anatomic snuffbox. The CT scan demonstrated radiographic union, and this was quantified using the method described by Singh et al. and judged to be approximately 83 % [10]. Therefore, based on the clinical and CT findings, the nonunion was judged to be united and the cast was removed for range of motion exercises. The patient was placed in a protective splint and instructed to begin passive and active range of motion exercises at the wrist with a gradual return to activity. He was asked to delay strength training until 10 weeks postoperatively.

The patient next returned to clinic 5 months postoperatively. He demonstrated excellent range of motion. Pronation and supi-

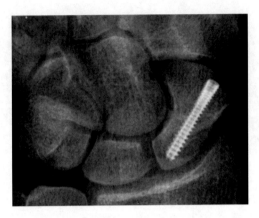

Fig. 7.7 PA X-ray of the left wrist at 5 months postoperatively demonstrating fracture union. (Published with kind permission of © Christopher Doherty and Ruby Grewal, 2015. All rights reserved)

nation were full. Extension and flexion at the wrist were 60° and 50°, respectively. Grip strength was 48 kg on the left side and 49 kg on the right. There was no pain at the wrist. The disabilities of the arm, shoulder and hand (DASH) and patient-rated wrist evaluation (PRWE) scores were both 0 (0 being the best possible score), indicating that he did not report any pain or disability. Figure 7.7 is an X-ray demonstrating excellent union across the waist of the scaphoid. The patient was advised to return to full activity without restriction.

At the 1-year follow-up, the patient reported no pain at the wrist with any limitations on his ability to play hockey. His wrist flexion was 75° and extension 80°. Grip strength on the left hand was 55 kg and that on the right was 60 kg.

Clinical Pearls/Pitfalls

• The most important step in deciding to proceed with internal fixation without bone graft is case selection. This decision should be based on clinical, radiographic, and intraoperative assessments. Clinically, the duration since injury is an important

factor to consider. Injuries in closer proximity to the procedure are more likely to have an opportunity to heal in comparison with those more remote from the procedure.
• Careful radiographic assessment is required to ensure that the fracture is minimally displaced across the waist of the scaphoid, without a significant humpback deformity and without evidence of AVN.

Intraoperative inspection is felt to be a key step in determining whether internal fixation alone is appropriate. This can be done arthroscopically or via an open volar approach based on the degree of suspicion that bone graft is required. It can be helpful to place a k-wire into the nonunion site intraoperatively to help identify the location of the fracture. In addition, we look for an intact cartilaginous cap as an indicator that bone grafting is not required (Fig. 7.4). It is important to be ready to bone graft if necessary; therefore, the patient should be consented and donor site prepared for this.

Literature Review and Discussion

Scaphoid nonunion is a nonhealing scaphoid fracture after 6 months of injury [11]. Nonoperative measures may be a consideration in the early course of treatment, particularly if the patient presents relatively close to the 6-month mark post-injury or if they have not had an appropriate course of immobilization. However, distinguishing between a delayed union (a fracture amenable to union with a course of immobilization) and a nonunion (which will require surgical fixation) can be difficult as there is little evidence in the literature to guide this decision. Percutaneous screw fixation has been described as an effective means to manage acute scaphoid waist fractures [12]. This philosophy has been extended to management of scaphoid waist nonunions that are nondisplaced and do not have evidence of significant sclerosis or bone loss at the fracture site [8]. Slade et al. studied 15 consecutive patients with scaphoid fibrous union or scaphoid nonunion without substantial sclerosis (less than 1 mm) treated with arthroscopically assisted percutaneous internal fixation without bone graft [8]. Arthroscopy was used to confirm fibrous union or an intact cartilaginous cap around a scaphoid nonunion. This study showed that all scaphoids went on to union at an average of 14 weeks postoperatively. The average range of motion was 49° extension and 61° flexion. Time to postoperative union was significantly increased as the time from injury to surgical intervention increased [8]. Prevention of micromotion at the fracture site is thought to be the key mechanism of healing with this technique in comparison with cast immobilization [8]. Saint-Cyr et al. presented their retrospective series of patients with delayed and nonunion of the scaphoid treated with dorsal percutaneous rigid fixation without bone graft [13]. They report a union rate of 100 % with no significant complications. The delayed union group had an earlier time to union (mean 7 weeks) versus the established nonunion group (mean 13 weeks). The average grip strength was 39 kg in the affected hand as compared to 45 kg in the unaffected hand [13]. Some authors have widened the indications for this technique. Mahmoud and Kapton presented a series of 27 consecutive patients who had nondisplaced scaphoid nonunions with substantial bone resorption (2 mm) treated with percutaneous internal fixation without bone graft [14]. They demonstrated that all fractures went on to union at a mean 11.6 weeks with an improvement in pain and range of motion [14]. Jeon et al. reported two cases of skeletally immature patients (aged 13 and 15 years) with scaphoid nonunions managed with percutaneous internal fixation [15]. Both cases went on to scaphoid union with good clinical outcomes. A percutaneous approach to internal fixation of scaphoid nonunions is a popular technique for accessing the scaphoid, but it can be technically demanding. Accurate guide wire and subsequent screw placement can be difficult. Careful examination of the intraoperative images is essential to ensure that the screw is not malpositioned or prominent. Complications of this approach must be considered. Bushnell et al. retrospectively reviewed 24 patients undergoing dorsal percutaneous cannulated screw fixation for acute undisplaced scaphoid waist fractures [16]. They report a major complication rate of 21 % (nonunion, hardware problems, and postoperative proximal pole fracture) and a minor complication rate of 8 % (intraoperative breakage of a cannulated screw and intraoperative breakage of a guide wire) [16]. These risks must be balanced against risks relevant to an open approach, such as soft tissue stripping, volar radiocarpal ligament division, neuroma, blood supply disruption, and scarring [13]. Scaphoid nonunion is a challenging problem for the surgeon. Several options exist for managing this condition. Patients with an undisplaced waist nonunion with minimal sclerosis and no change in the architecture of the scaphoid can be considered for rigid internal fixation without bone grafting. We present a case demonstrating that this technique is effective at establishing union with good clinical outcomes and early return to activity.

References

1. Temple CL, Ross DC, Bennett JD, Garvin GJ, King Gj, Faber KJ. Comparison of sagittal computed tomography and plain film radiography in a scaphoid fracture model. J Hand Surg (Am). 2005;30A:534–42.
2. Lozano-Calderon S, Blazar P, Zurakowski D, Lee SG, Ring D. Diagnosis of scaphoid fracture displacement with radiography and computed tomography. J Bone Jt Surg. 2006;88A:2695–703.
3. Schmitt R, Heinze A, Fellner F, et al. Imaging and staging of avascular osteonecroses at the wrist and hand. Eur J Radiol. 1997;25:92–103.
4. Kawamura K, Chung KC. Treatment of scaphoid fractures and nonunions. J Hand Surg (Am). 2008;33A:988–97.
5. Osterman AL, Mikulics M. Scaphoid nonunion. Hand Clin. 1988;4:437–55.
6. Capo JT, Orillaza NS Jr, Slade JF 3rd. Percutaneous management of scaphoid nonunions. Tech Hand Up Extrem Surg. 2009;13(1):23–29.
7. Barton NJ. Apparent and partial non-union of the scaphoid. J Hand Surg (Br). 1996;21B(4):496–500.
8. Slade JF, Geissler WB, Gutow AP, et al. Percutaneous internal fixation of selected scaphoid nonunions with an arthroscopically assisted dorsal approach. J Bone Jt Surg. 2003;85A(4):20–32.
9. Buijze GA, Ochtman L, Ring D. Management of scaphoid nonunions. J Hand Surg (Am.). 2012;37A:1095–100.
10. Singh HP, Forward D, Davis TRC, et al. Partial union of acute scaphoid fractures. J Hand Surg (Br). 2005;30:440–5.
11. Trumble TE, Salas P, Barthell T et al. Management of scaphoid nonunions. J Am Acad Orthop Surg. 2003;11:380–91.

12. McQueen MM, Gelbke MK, Wakefield A, et al. Percutaneous screw fixation versus conservative treatment for fractures of the waist of the scaphoid. J Bone Jt Surg (Br). 2008;90B: 66–71.

13. Saint-Cyr M, Oni G, Wong C, et al. Dorsal percutaneous cannulated screw fixation for delayed union and nonunion of the scaphoid. Plastic Reconstruct Surg. 2011;128:467–73.

14. Mahmoud M, Koptan W. Percutaneous screw fixation without bone grafting for established scaphoid nonunion with substantial bone loss. J Bone Jt Surg (Br). 2011;93B:932–6.

15. Jeon I, Kochhar H, Lee B, et al. Percutaneous screw fixation for scaphoid nonunion in skeletally immature patients: a report of two cases. J Hand Surg. 2008;33A:656–9.

16. Bushnell BD, McWilliams AD, Messer TM. Complications in dorsal cannulated screw fixation of nondisplaced scaphoid waist fractures. J Hand Surg. 2007;32A:827–33.

Chapter 8
Scaphoid Nonunion Open Treatment with Distal Radius Bone Graft via Mini Dorsal Approach

Michael Lin and Tamara D. Rozental

Case Presentation

A 26-year-old right-hand-dominant male presented for evaluation for right wrist pain. He sustained a fall during a volleyball match 4-months prior and continued to experience significant wrist pain during the activities of daily living. Limitations included the inability to lift heavy objects.

Physical Examination

The patient exhibited no swelling or deformity. He had no pain over the distal radius or ulna but had pain in the anatomic snuffbox. He had wrist motion of 45° of extension and 40° of flexion, whereas his contralateral wrist had 65° of flexion and extension. He had full forearm rotation, and full digital motion bilaterally.

T. D. Rozental (✉)
Department of Orthopaedic Surgery, Beth Israel Deaconess Medical Center, Harvard Medical School, Boston, MA, USA
e-mail: trozenta@bidmc.harvard.edu

M. Lin
Alpine Orthopaedic Medical Group, Inc, Stockton, CA, USA

© Springer International Publishing Switzerland 2015
J. Yao (ed.), *Scaphoid Fractures and Nonunions*,
DOI 10.1007/978-3-319-18977-2_8

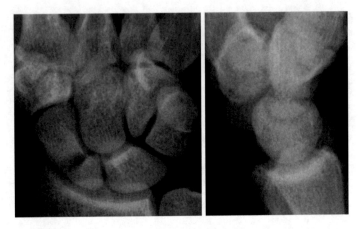

Fig. 8.1 Preoperative X-ray showing scaphoid nonunion with cystic defect. (Published with kind permission of © Michael Lin and Tamara D. Rozental, 2015. All Rights Reserved.)

Diagnostic Testing

AP, lateral, and oblique X-rays of the wrist showed a nonunion through the proximal third of the scaphoid with cystic changes (Fig. 8.1). CT scan of the wrist was obtained to determine whether a humpback deformity was present. The CT revealed a distracted fracture with minimal bony contact but without dorsal osteophyte or humpback deformity (Fig. 8.2).

Because of the patient's young age and potential risk for degenerative arthritis, surgical treatment was discussed. Given the lack of humpback deformity, the decision was made to proceed with open reduction internal fixation with cancellous bone grafting through a dorsal approach.

Surgical Technique

Surgery is performed under regional nerve block and MAC anesthesia. Prophylactic antibiotics are given prior to incision. After exsanguinating the forearm, a 2-cm incision is made just ulnar to

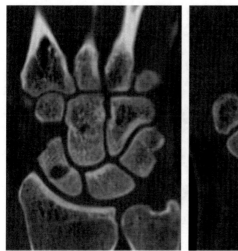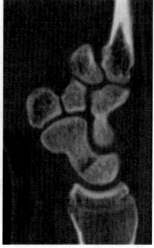

Fig. 8.2 Representative slices of preoperative CT demonstrating scaphoid nonunion with cystic defect. Notice there is no humpback deformity. (Published with kind permission of © Michael Lin and Tamara D. Rozental, 2015. All Rights Reserved.)

Lister's tubercle. The extensor retinaculum is incised over the third dorsal compartment, and the EPL tendon is retracted radially. A distal radius cortical bone window proximal to Lister's tubercle is created, and 1 mL of cancellous bone graft is harvested. The cortical window is replaced after bone graft harvest. A 1-cm longitudinal incision is then made in the dorsal proximal capsule. The wrist is brought into hyperflexion until the proximal pole of the scaphoid is visualized. In this patient, a guidewire from the Acutrak 2 (Hillsboro, OR) mini screw set was advanced from proximal to distal in a central position in both the AP and lateral planes. Once the position was confirmed radiographically, a second anti-rotation guidewire was placed. The central guidewire was over-drilled and removed. The distal radius cancellous bone graft was then packed through the drill hole into the nonunion site.

After bone grafting, the central guidewire was replaced, and the position was confirmed radiographically to ensure that the wire was in the proper path. An Acutrak 2 mini screw was then advanced

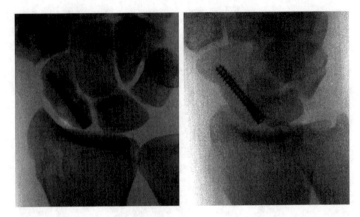

Fig. 8.3 Intraoperative fluoroscopy demonstrating bone graft of cystic defect, proper screw placement, and fracture compression. (Published with kind permission of © Michael Lin and Tamara D. Rozental, 2015. All Rights Reserved.)

over the wire to achieve fixation and compression of the fracture. AP, lateral and oblique fluoroscopic images were taken to confirm proper screw position (Fig. 8.3). After wound irrigation, the capsule and the extensor retinaculum were repaired. The subcutaneous tissue and skin were closed with Monocryl, followed by Steri-Strips. A thumb spica splint was applied.

Clinical Course and Outcome

The patient was brought back to the office in 10 days for application of a short arm thumb spica cast. Radiographs were obtained on the first postoperative visit to confirm adequate positioning of the hardware. At 2 months, a CT scan of the wrist was obtained to assess fracture healing and showed early bony bridging. The patient was placed in a second thumb spica cast. A second CT scan at 4 months demonstrated obvious fracture healing (Fig. 8.4). At this point, the patient was transitioned to a splint and began occupation therapy for range of motion and strengthening exercises. At final follow-up 8 months after surgery (Fig. 8.5), the patient

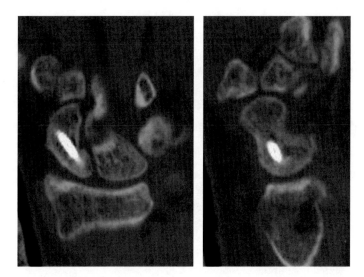

Fig. 8.4 Postoperative CT at 4 months showing definitive fracture healing. Note the visible bone graft donor site. (Published with kind permission of © Michael Lin and Tamara D. Rozental, 2015. All Rights Reserved.)

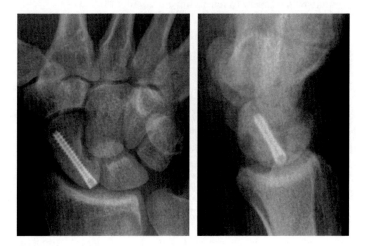

Fig. 8.5 Final follow-up X-ray at 8 months demonstrating fracture healing and complete resolution of cystic defect. (Published with kind permission of © Michael Lin and Tamara D. Rozental, 2015. All Rights Reserved.)

exhibited wrist extension of 58°, flexion of 63°, radial deviation of 15°, and ulnar deviation 20°. His grip strength was 104 lbs compared to 120 lbs in the contralateral side. He reported no limitations in activities and had a quickDASH score of 2.3.

Clinical Pearls and Pitfalls

- Obtain a preoperative CT scan to determine whether a humpback deformity is present. If a deformity exists, structural bone graft may be more appropriate.
- Place the incision just ulnar to Lister's tubercle and protect the EPL tendon.
- Place the wrist in hyperflexion to allow visualization of the proximal pole of the scaphoid.
- Obtain fluoroscopic images with the wrist in slight flexion to avoid bending the guide wires as the wrist is extended.
- Following the removal of the guide wire for bone graft insertion, it may be necessary to redrill the tract before replacing the guide wire and compression screw.
- Obtain a postoperative CT scan to adequately assess for healing

Literature Review and Discussion

Neglected scaphoid nonunion predictably results in pain and functional impairment; and can lead to scaphoid humpback deformity, radiocarpal arthrosis, and eventual advanced carpal collapse [1–3]. Therefore, with the exception of the elderly or poor surgical candidates, we typically recommend surgical treatment to achieve fracture union. The technique presented here is ideal for early scaphoid nonunion without extensive sclerosis or significant alteration in the overall scaphoid geometry. Cases of significant osteonecrosis may be better addressed with vascularized bone graft [4–6], and patients with shortened scaphoid or humpback deformity are better served by corticocancellous graft to restore proper scaphoid anatomy.[7, 8] As illustrated in this case presentation, our technique reliably and effectively treats scaphoid nonunion with cystic defect without the need for extensive open debridement or bone grafting. Perhaps some of the success is attributable to a limited dorsal approach which minimizes the disruption of the scaphoid's external blood supply by preserving the dorsal radial and anterior interosseous arterial branches of radial artery and the anterior interosseous artery [9]. We routinely educate patients on the tenuous nature of scaphoid's vascular supply and the possibility of delayed healing despite optimal surgical technique. Additionally, we feel that postoperative cast treatment and CT evaluation of healing is an important component of this treatment protocol. All of our patients received short arm thumb spica cast postoperatively for at least 2 months, with subsequent CT evaluation. The cast is discontinued after radiological evidence of union.

References

1. Mack GR, et al. The natural history of scaphoid nonunion. J Bone Joint Surg Am. 1984;66:504–9.
2. Ruby LK, Stinson J, Belsky MR. The natural history of scaphoid nonunion. A review of 55 cases. J Bone Joint Surg AM. 1985;67:428–32.
3. Kosin SH. Incidence, mechanism, and natural history of scaphoid fractures. Hand Clin. 2001;17:515–24.
4. Straw RG, et al. Scaphoid nonunion: treatment with a pedicled vascularized bone graft based on the 1–2 intercompartmental supraretinacular branch of the radial artery. J. Hand Surg. 2002;27B:413.
5. Sotereanos DG, et al. A capsular-based vascularized distal radius graft for proximal scaphoid pseudoarthrosis. J. Hand Surg. 2006;31(4):508–7.
6. Jones DB, et al. Free-vascularized medial femoral condyle transfer in the treatment of scaphoid nonunions. Plast Reconstr Surg 2010;125:1176–84.
7. Fernandez DL. A technique for anterior wedge-shaped grafts for scaphoid nonunions with carpal instability. J Hand Surg. 1984;9(5):733–7.
8. Hanel DP, Kim PS. Carpus: nonunion and Malunion. In ASSH Textbook of Hand and Upper Extremity Surgery. 2013;1:269–81.
9. Gelberman RH, Menon J. The vascularity of the scaphoid bone. J Hand Surg AM. 1980;5(5):508–13.

Chapter 9
Scaphoid Nonunion: Surgical Fixation with Local Nonvascularized Bone Graft (Open)

Sidney M. Jacoby and Justin D. Stull

Case Presentation

A healthy, 20-year-old right-hand dominant collegiate student athlete presented with a chief complaint of persistent left wrist pain. Three months prior to his presentation, the patient recalled falling awkwardly and landing on an outstretched and hyperextended left wrist during a sporting event. The patient reported persistent pain and limited wrist range of motion, particularly in dorsiflexion.

Physical Assessment

On physical examination, the patient was in mild distress secondary to left wrist discomfort. He was otherwise a well developed and healthy individual standing 190 cm tall and weighing 88 kg.

S. M. Jacoby (✉)
Department of Orthopaedic Surgery, Thomas Jefferson University Hospital,
The Franklin Suite G114, 834 Chestnut St., Philadelphia, PA, USA
e-mail: smjacoby@handcenters.com

J. D. Stull
Sidney Kimmel Medical College at Thomas Jefferson University,
Philadelphia, PA, USA
e-mail: Justin.stull@gmail.com

© Springer International Publishing Switzerland 2015
J. Yao (ed.), *Scaphoid Fractures and Nonunions*,
DOI 10.1007/978-3-319-18977-2_9

Neck, shoulder, elbow, and digital range of motion were equal, symmetric, and painless.

Focal evaluation of the patient's left wrist revealed pain in the anatomic snuffbox and pain with scaphoid shift test. While there was no appreciable swelling compared to the contralateral uninjured wrist, the patient had limited range of motion in his left wrist with extension 50° (vs. 75°) and flexion 60° (vs. 70°).

Diagnostic Studies

Radiographs performed during the first evaluation (6 months following the initial trauma) revealed a scaphoid waist fracture with lucency and cystic changes suggestive of an early nonunion. Lateral projections revealed a humpback deformity with no scapholunate interval widening. Computed tomography (CT) confirmed the scaphoid nonunion and thin cuts through the plane of the scaphoid further verified collapse indicative of an early humpback deformity at the scaphoid mid-waist nonunion as shown in Fig. 9.1.

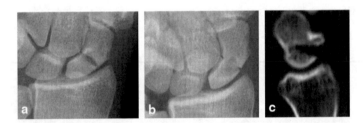

Fig. 9.1 Preoperative imaging. **a** The scaphoid nonunion is clearly noted on the standard PA wrist radiograph. **b** The scaphoid waist view reveals cystic changes consistent with nonunion. **c** Sagittal CT imaging of the humpback deformity. This image shows the classic humpback deformity as angulation of opposing poles of the scaphoid in the presence of a mid-waist nonunion. (Published with kind permission of © Sidney M. Jacoby and Justin D. Stull, 2015. All rights reserved)

Diagnosis

Scaphoid waist nonunion with humpback deformity

Management Options

Management options for scaphoid nonunion are based on a number of factors including the location of the fracture, vascularity, the degree of carpal instability, and a critical analysis of early degenerative changes. In this case, the patient is a healthy college athlete with a mid-waist scaphoid nonunion showing early signs of a humpback deformity. We consider numerous variables in formulating a treatment plan including: (1) timing of intervention, (2) choice of procedure, (3) surgical approach, (4) graft donor location, and (5) method of fixation.

In the setting of scaphoid nonunion with humpback deformity, surgical intervention is necessary both to correct scaphoid geometry and to promote healing via internal fixation. If left untreated, collapse of the scaphoid waist due to deterioration of the lesion's opposing ends can further deteriorate into dorsal intercalated segment instability (DISI) [1–3]. Eventually, failure to achieve union will result in a predictable pattern of scaphoid nonunion advanced collapse (SNAC) with additional long-term sequelae. While nonoperative treatment may be utilized for acute nondisplaced scaphoid fractures, in the setting of a known scaphoid nonunion, particularly those with carpal collapse, nonoperative treatment is considered suboptimal [4].

Selection of operative technique should be based primarily on the location of the scaphoid fracture and the vascular integrity of the proximal pole. While a dorsal approach is typically utilized for proximal pole fractures, in the setting of a scaphoid nonunion at the waist or distal pole, a volar approach spares the dorsal blood supply. This blood supply is received at the dorsal ridge of the scaphoid and provides arterial inflow to 70–80 % of the bone, including the proximal pole [3, 5, 6]. Additionally, as is the case in this particular patient's fracture pattern, humpback deformities necessitate volar access to facilitate secure fixation of the graft and the internal fixation device [5, 7].

A critical consideration in scaphoid nonunion surgery is the potential need for a vascularized bone graft to address scaphoid avascular necrosis (AVN). In the setting of AVN, both the osseous nonunion and the vascular status can be addressed with a vascularized bone graft and internal fixation [8, 9]. However, in the absence of AVN, there is a diminished indication for a vascularized bone graft, and nonvascularized bone graft is acceptable [1, 10].

With the decision to utilize an avascular graft, various donor graft sites are considered, including the distal radius, iliac crest, medial proximal tibia, and olecranon [11]. The iliac crest is distinguished for both its strength and pluripotent stem cells [12], while distal radius bone grafting offers the advantage of proximity to the implantation site, thus potentially reducing surgical morbidity associated with choosing a donor site ectopic to the scaphoid incision [13, 14]. In a comparison between iliac bone grafts and those derived from the distal radius, it has been reported that the source of graft donor site does not have a significant impact on the healing and incorporation of the graft [3, 14, 15].

Preference for a wedge graft over cancellous autograft bone is indicated to properly correct scaphoid collapse associated with a humpback deformity [7, 16]. The wedge graft utilizes a corticocancellous graft with additional cancellous bone to augment the recipient site [17].

Management Chosen

The patient presented in this report was a healthy young male, with radiographic evidence of scaphoid nonunion with humpback deformity and no radiographic evidence of AVN. The decision was made to proceed with a wedge-shaped nonvascularized distal radial bone graft to correct the scaphoid nonunion and associated humpback deformity. Fixation with a cannulated, continuous headless compression screw via a volar approach was also utilized.

Operative Technique

Following routine prep and drape as well as administration of IV antibiotics, the limb was elevated, and tourniquet inflated. A modified Russe approach was utilized extending from the distal volar radial forearm, paralleling the thenar web space [18, 19]. The flexor carpi radialis tendon was incised along its ulnar margin and the subsheath was identified and released. Blunt dissection was performed in order to mobilize the forearm flexors, and the thenar musculature was gently elevated in order to gain access to the distal pole of the scaphoid. In a capsular sparing approach popularized by Garcia-Elias [20], a "U-shaped" incision was made directly over the scaphoid and extended proximally along the radial aspect of the radial metaphysis (Fig. 9.2). The distal pole and the body of the scaphoid were identified with the use of intraoperative fluoroscopic imaging and an 18-gauge needle. Intraoperatively, the scaphoid nonunion demonstrated a humpback deformity that had previously been visualized on CT imaging. K-wires were then placed in the proximal and distal scaphoid poles in a position that would later allow for optimal positioning of a guidewire for the

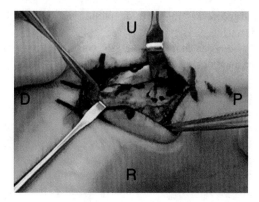

Fig. 9.2 Volar capsular ligament splitting approach to the scaphoid. This approach minimizes trauma to the capsule, while allowing for appropriate visualization of the scaphoid and distal radius. *D* distal, *P* proximal, *R* radial, *U* ulnar. (Published with kind permission of © Sidney M. Jacoby and Justin D. Stull, 2015. All rights reserved)

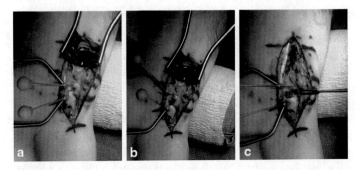

Fig. 9.3 Intraoperative visualization of the scaphoid nonunion. **a** Placement of K-wires for the small bone distractor. Note that the distractor is placed in a location that will not interfere with later guidewire placement for scaphoid screw. **b** Pre-graft distraction of nonunion site and debridement of nonunion in preparation for cancellous and cortico-cancellous graft. **c** Post-wedge graft placement in the mid-waist of the scaphoid nonunion, providing correction of the humpback deformity. Note that the distractor is no longer utilized to provide a distraction force and will be removed prior to scaphoid screw insertion. (Published with kind permission of © Sidney M. Jacoby and Justin D. Stull, 2015. All rights reserved)

fixation screw. A small bone distractor was positioned around the K-wires and utilized to maintain distraction during this portion of the procedure (Fig. 9.3).

It should be noted that the distractor was later removed during screw fixation. If desired, a compressor bone clamp can be applied in its place during screw insertion to maintain compression.

The fracture site was identified and all fibrous debris within the nonunion site was carefully debrided with a combination of small curettes and a small burr. Throughout this delicate process, irrigation was utilized to minimize the risk of heat necrosis to the scaphoid. Importantly, the proximal pole of the scaphoid was noted to have punctate bleeding when the tourniquet was released indicating adequate vascularity. Direct measurement revealed an 8-mm gap at the nonunion site. The fracture fragments were mobilized with the previously placed K-wires and an appropriately sized graft harvested from the volar distal radius.

To access the volar distal radius, the pronator quadratus was gently elevated, and a 1-cm^2 graft was chosen. A K-wire was utilized to mark the borders of the distal radius bone graft. To obtain a rectangular-shaped corticocancellous bone graft, an osteotome and mallet were utilized. Cancellous bone was also harvested from the volar distal radius donor site.

Attention was directed back to the scaphoid nonunion site, where a small amount of harvested cancellous graft was packed into the void created by the scaphoid nonunion. At this stage, the volar distal radius corticocancellous graft was sculpted and wedged into the scaphoid nonunion site with gentle distraction provided by the previously placed small bone clamp distractor in order to recreate the normal intra-scaphoid angle.

Intraoperative fluoroscopy revealed correction of the humpback deformity with placement of an appropriately sized graft into the scaphoid nonunion site. A guidewire was placed down the central axis of the scaphoid to stabilize the graft. Upon measurement, a 24-mm scaphoid screw was deemed to be the appropriate size. To minimize migration of the graft, as well as to minimize heat necrosis to the scaphoid, reaming for the screw was performed by hand. At this point, a 24-mm, headless Acutrak II (Acumed, Hillsboro, OR) screw was inserted in a retrograde fashion. There was an excellent fixation noted with compression across the scaphoid nonunion site. Intraoperative fluoroscopy demonstrated appropriate placement of the screw in multiple planes. Crushed cancellous bone allograft was then placed into the void at the donor site at the volar distal radius and the pronator quadratus was gently repaired over the volar distal radius. The volar capsule and subcutaneous tissue were repaired with 3-0 Vicryl with 4-0 Nylon used to close the skin. Sterile dressings were applied, including a short-arm thumb spica splint.

Clinical Course and Outcome

The patient presented back to the clinic 6 days postoperatively for the first evaluation. Radiographic imaging demonstrated a well-positioned bone graft and fixation of the scaphoid waist fracture with the surgical screw in a near center–center position on multiple views. There was evidence of an improved intra-scaphoid angle indicative of correction of the previous humpback deformity.

At 1 month postoperatively, the patient had well-healed surgical incisions, marked improvement in swelling, and less pain in the anatomic snuffbox with deep palpation. Range of motion revealed 30° extension and 30° flexion with full digital range of motion. Radiographic imaging showed evidence of scaphoid healing, indicating a well-incorporated bone graft and fixation of the scaphoid waist fracture with the compression screw still in unchanged position on multiple views. A scaphoid mobilization splint was provided, allowing for gentle range of motion, including "dart throwers" motion. The scaphoid mobilization splint is a dynamic splint that offers limited wrist motion, but at the same time allows for direction-specific range of motion. In this case, radial and ulnar deviation with limited flexion and extension was allowed. The scaphoid mobilization splint provides the ability to mildly stretch the soft tissues of the wrist including the joint capsule, potentially minimizing postoperative contractures. A certified hand therapist provided instruction and guidance throughout the postoperative therapy.

At two months postoperatively, the patient presented with minimal pain in the anatomical snuffbox and little residual swelling of the operative wrist. He noted mild stiffness on wrist extension with a painless arc of motion between 20° extension and 40° flexion. With compliant splint use, stiffness and early limitations in range of motion were to be expected. CT imaging showed proper screw alignment and fixation with central osseous fusion indicating progressive healing. At this point, the patient was progressed to full range of motion, which was encouraged under direct supervision of a certified hand therapist.

At 3 months postoperatively, the splint was discontinued and the patient was returned to uninhibited mobilization. At 4 months, the patient was cleared for weight lifting within tolerance. Throughout the rehabilitation process, the patient was instructed to discontinue range of motion or rehabilitation exercise with any pain.

At 20 weeks postoperatively, physical examination revealed minimal discomfort on palpation of the anatomical snuffbox. Wrist extension measured 60°, flexion 55°, radial deviation 10°, and ulnar deviation 20°, all of which were performed without pain. Grip strength was the only lasting deficit with the left-hand grip strength of 70 lbs compared to 120 lbs with the right hand. CT imaging revealed progressive healing with proper scaphoid align-

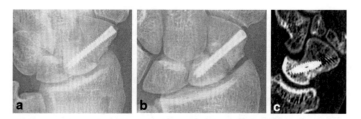

Fig. 9.4 Postoperative imaging. **a** and **b** One month postoperative radiographs. Follow-up studies revealed screw placement through the central axis of the scaphoid in two distinct planes with evidence of progressive union. **c** Sagittal CT imaging of corrected humpback deformity at 2 months postoperative. Follow-up imaging displays the screw placement through the scaphoid correcting the previous humpback deformity with evidence of bony trabeculae crossing the previous nonunion site. (Published with kind permission of © Sidney M. Jacoby and Justin D. Stull, 2015. All rights reserved)

ment, screw position, and near complete osseous union (Fig. 9.4). Return to tolerable athletic activity was deemed appropriate at this point in the patient's recovery.

Clinical Pearls/Pitfalls

- Elevate, but do not exsanguinate the limb prior to tourniquet inflation to be able to visualize potential vessels for vascularized bone grafting if necessary and to be able to evaluate for punctate bleeding at the nonunion site.
- Volar capsular ligament splitting approach is made to help minimize the risk of capsular contracture, perhaps improving wrist extension range of motion.
- Use a distractor/compressor bone clamp applied to K-wires placed in the scaphoid (Fig. 9.2). This helps in distracting the fracture fragments to adequately debride the nonunion and pack cortico-cancellous graft into the depth of the scaphoid cavity.
- Intraoperative assessment of proximal pole punctate bleeding is critical to evaluate adequate proximal scaphoid vascularity. In the absence of punctate bleeding, strong consideration should be given to a vascularized bone graft.

- Compression screw fixation is the typical method of choice with consideration of temporary scapho-capitate pinning, to minimize stress across the nonunion site.

Literature Review and Discussion

The management of scaphoid fractures, and nonunions in particular, remains a challenging issue for both the patient and provider. With prompt diagnosis, nonoperative treatment can be considered for a limited number of scaphoid fracture patterns. Diligent and consistent immobilization may be difficult to achieve and in the case of physical laborers, care providers or athletes, prolonged immobilization may not be a realistic option. Additional risk factors such as scaphoid nonunion, scaphoid collapse, and signs of AVN are clear indications for operative intervention due to the poor healing potential and the inevitable pattern of degenerative wrist arthrosis known as SNAC wrist.

Surgical correction of scaphoid nonunions utilizing open reduction with bone grafting was first discussed in the literature in 1928 [21]. Initial discussion centered around the optimal surgical approach as well as graft harvest location, and by 1935, it was reported that bone grafting resulted in improved outcomes as compared to prolonged immobilization or scaphoidectomy [21–23]. Matti et al. proposed an inlay bone graft via a dorsal approach to more closely approximate native scaphoid anatomy. In 1960, Russe described a palmar approach for the formation of the bone cavity, and filling of the cavity with cortical and cancellous autograft harvested from the iliac crest. The technique of filling the nonunion area with cortical and cancellous autograft through a palmar approach is referred to as Matti–Russe technique, which for many years was the standard treatment of scaphoid nonunions [24–27]. Most major innovations, since Russe published his technique in 1960, have been in the realm of securing fracture compression with rigid internal fixation. McLaughlin first proposed screw fixation for scaphoid nonunion in 1953 [28]. In 1984, Herbert introduced a variable pitch screw to improve compression across the nonunion, and thus successful rates of correction for scaphoid nonunions

[29]. Since then, numerous implant manufacturers have contributed to the current generation of cannulated, variable pitch screws offering even greater compression across the nonunion site, as demonstrated by numerous biomechanical studies. Kirschner wires (K-wires) have been used with some success. However, they do not provide the compression forces that can be achieved with variable pitch screw fixation, and are better reserved for supportive immobilization with compression screw fixation [30–33].

Another critical element in treating scaphoid nonunions is close evaluation of vascular integrity at the scaphoid proximal pole. On advanced MRI, avascularity may be identified by an increase in signal intensity between the nonunion surfaces with decreased signal intensity throughout the nonperfused bone [34, 35]. Intraoperative punctate bleeding is of critical importance in the final selection of donor graft site, yielding better predictability than MRI or any other nonoperative imaging techniques and one should always be prepared to harvest vascularized bone graft should intraoperative findings dictate [1]. Another small pearl that we have incorporated within all scaphoid nonunion cases is to elevate, but not exsanguinate the limb prior to tourniquet inflation. In the case presented in this chapter, intraoperative findings revealed appropriate punctate bleeding, and thus the preoperative decision to utilize a nonvascularized distal radius bone graft was validated.

In summary, in the setting of scaphoid nonunion with humpback deformity and no evidence of AVN at the proximal pole, nonvascularized distal radius bone grafting with screw fixation can be considered an effective treatment option to correct scaphoid deformity, and achieve osseous union with the expectation of good long-term results. Adherence to sound surgical principles and appropriate postoperative immobilization with close radiographic follow-up are all contributing factors to success.

References

1. Kawamura K, Chung K. Treatment of scaphoid fractures and nonunions. J Hand Surg 2008;33A:988–97.
2. Langhoff O, Andersen JL. Consequences of late immobilization of scaphoid fractures. J Hand Surg [Br]. 1988;13:77–9.

3. Schuind F, Haentjens P, Van Innis F, Vander Maren C, Garcia-Elias M, Sennwald G. Prognostic factors in the treatment of carpal scaphoid nonunions. J Hand Surg. 1999;24A:761–76.

4. Ruby L, Stinson J, Belsky M. The natural history of scaphoid non-union: a review of fifty-five cases. J Bone Jt Surg. 1985;67-A:428–32.

5. Gelberman R, Menon J. The vascularity of the scaphoid bone. J Hand Surg. 1980;5:508–13.

6. Waitayawinyu T, McCallister WV, Nemechek NM, Trumble TE. Surgical techniques: scaphoid nonunion. J Am Acad Orhop Surg. 2007;15:308–20.

7. Bindra R, Bednar M, Light T. Volar wedge grafting for scaphoid nonunion with collapse. J Hand Surg. 2008:33A:974–9.

8. Ribak S, Medina C, Mattar R, Ulson H, de Resende M, Etchebehere M. Treatment of scaphoid nonunion with vascularized and nonvascularized dorsal bone grafting from the distal radius. Int Orthop. 2010;34:683–8.

9. Green DP. The effect of avascular necrosis on russe bone grafting for scaphoid nonunion. J Hand Surg. 1985;10A:597–605.

10. Braga-Silva J, Peruchi FM, Moschen GM, Gehlen D, Padoin AV. A comparison of the use of distal radius vascularized bone graft and non-vascularized iliac crest bone graft in the treatment of non-union of scaphoid fractures. J Hand Surg. 2008;33E:636–40.

11. Bruno RJ, Cohen MS, Berzins A, Sumner DR. Bone graft harvesting from the distal radius, olecranon, and iliac crest: a quantitative analysis. J Hand Surg. 2001;26A:135–41.

12. Fisk GR. Volar wedge grafting of the carpal scaphoid in non-union associated with dorsal instability patterns (discussion). proceedings of seventh combined meeting of the orthopaedic associations of the english speaking world, Cape Town, South Africa, March, 1982. J Bone JT Surg [Br]. 1982;64:632–3.

13. Andrews J, Miller G, Haddad R. Treatment of scaphoid nonunion by volar inlay distal radius bone graft. J Hand Surg. 1985;10B:214–6.

14. Goyal T, Sankineani SR, Tripathy SK. Local distal radius bone graft versus iliac crest bone graft for scaphoid nonunion: a comparative study. Musculoskelet Surg. 2013;97(2):109–14.

15. Tambe AD, Cutler L, Stilwell J, Murali SR, Trail IA, Stanley JK. Scaphoid non-union: the role of vascularized grafting in recalcitrant non-unions of the scaphoid. J Hand Surg. 2006;31B:185–190.

16. Merrell GA, Wolfe SW, Slade JF III. Treatment of scaphoid nonunions: quantitative meta-analysis of the literature. J Hand Surg. 2002;27A:685–91.

17. Monreal R. Treatment of scaphoid nonunions with closed-wedge osteotomy of the distal radius: report of six cases. Hand. 2008;3:91–5.

18. Russe O. Fracture of the carpal navicular. Diagnosis, non-operative treatment, and operative treatment. J Bone Jt Surg. 1960;42A:759–68.

19. Zoubos AB, Triantafyllopoulos IK, Babis GC, Soucacos PN. Modified matti-russe technique for the treatment of scaphoid waist non-union and pseudoarthrosis. Med Sci Monit. 2011;17(2):MT7–12.

20. Hagert, E, Ferreres A, Garcia-Elias M. Nerve-sparing dorsal and volar approaches to the radiocarpal joint. J Hand Surg. 2010;35(7):1070–4.

21. Adams JD, Leonard RD. Fracture of the carpal scaphoid. N Engl J Med. 1928;198:401–4.

22. Sutro CJ. Treatment of nonunion of the carpal navicular bone. Surgery. 1946;20:536–40.

23. Murray G. End results of bone-grafting for non-union of the carpal navicular. J Bone JT Surg. 1946;28:749–56.

24. Matti H. Uber die behandling der navicularefraktur und der refractura patellae durch plombierung mit spongiosa. Zentralbl Chir. 1937;64:2353–9.

25. Moon ES, Dy CJ, Derman P, Vance MC, Carlson MG. Management of nonunion following surgical management of scaphoid fractures: current concepts. J Am Acad Orthop Surg. 2013;21:548–57.

26. Buijze GA, Ochtman L, Ring D. Management of scaphoid nonunion. J Hand Surg. 2012;37A:1095–100.

27. Sayegh ET, Strauch RJ. Graft choice in the management of unstable scaphoid nonunion: a systematic review. J Hand Surg. 2014;39:1500–1506e.

28. McLaughlin HL. Fracture of the carpal navicular bone: some observations based on treatment by open reduction and internal fixation. J Bone JT Surg. 1954;36-A:765–74.

29. Herbert TJ, Fisher WE. Management of the fractured scaphoid using a new bone screw. J Bone JT Surg Br. 1984;66B:114–23.

30. Lim TK, Kim HK, Koh KH, Lee HI, Woo SJ, Park MJ. Treatment of avascular proximal pole scaphoid nonunions with vascularized distal radius bone grafting. J Hand Surg. 2013;38A:1906–12e1.

31. Panchal A, Kubiak EN, Keshner M, Fulkerson E, Paksima N. Comparison of fixation methods for scaphoid nonunions. Bull NYU Hosp Jt Dis. 2007;65:271–5.

32. Jeon IH, Kochhar H, Lee BW, Kim SY, Kim PT. Percutaneous screw fixation for scaphoid nonunion in skeletal immature patients: a report of two cases. J Hand Surg. 2008;33A:656–9.

33. Daly KD, Gill P, Magnussen PA, Simonis RB. Established nonunion of the scaphoid treated by volar wedge grafting and herbert screw fixation. J Bone JT Surg [Br]. 1996;78B:530–4.

34. Geissler WB, Slade JF. Fractures of the Carpal Bones. In Wolf SW, Pederson WC, Hotchkiss RN, Kozin SH, Cohen MS, eds. Green's Operative Hand Surgery. Sixth Edition, Philadephia, PA: Churchill Livingstone; 2011:639–707.

35. Trumble TE. Avascular Necrosis After Scaphoid Fracture: A correlation of magnetic resonance imaging and histology. J Hand Surg Am. 1990;15:557–64.

Suggested Readings

Braga-Silva. A comparison of the use of distal radius vascularized bone graft and non-vascularized iliac crest bone graft in the treatment of non-union of scaphoid fractures. J Hand Surg. 2008;33E:636–40.

Goyal T, Sankineani SR, Tripathy SK. Local distal radius bone graft versus iliac crest bone graft for scaphoid nonunion: a comparative study. Musculo-skelet Surg. 2013;97(2):109–14.

Chapter 10
Scaphoid Nonunion Treated with Iliac Crest Structural Autograft

Roberto Diaz and James Chang

Case Presentation

A healthy 22-year-old right-hand dominant professional mountain biker sustained a left scaphoid waist fracture after a fall from his mountain bike. He initially presented to an outside hospital where he was treated with cast immobilization for 4 weeks. He went on to develop a scaphoid nonunion that was subsequently treated with open reduction and internal fixation using distal radius bone graft. He presented 2 years after his injury with persistent radial-sided wrist pain limiting his ability to ride his bicycle competitively. There is no relevant past medical history and the patient denied tobacco use.

R. Diaz (✉)
Department of Orthopaedic Surgery, Stanford University, 450 Broadway, Redwood City, CA 94063, USA
e-mail: ridiaz@stanford.edu

J. Chang
Division of Plastic and Reconstructive Surgery, Department of Orthopaedics, Stanford School of Medicine, 450 Broadway St., Pavilion A 2nd Fl MC 6120, Redwood City, CA 94063, USA
e-mail: jameschang@stanford.edu

© Springer International Publishing Switzerland 2015
J. Yao (ed.), *Scaphoid Fractures and Nonunions*,
DOI 10.1007/978-3-319-18977-2_10

Physical Assessment

Physical examination revealed 85° of wrist flexion, 75° of wrist extension, and full supination/pronation. In addition, there was tenderness along the anatomic snuffbox and at the scaphoid tubercle.

Diagnostic Studies

The evaluation of a patient with wrist pain begins with a complete history and physical along with radiographic imaging consisting of a wrist PA, oblique, lateral, and a scaphoid view. Radiographs obtained at the patient's initial visit revealed bone resorption at the fracture site and lucency surrounding the compression screw, findings consistent with a scaphoid nonunion (Fig. 10.1, 10.2). Mild radial styloid beaking was noted on the AP radiograph indicating early stages of a stage I scaphoid nonunion advanced collapse (SNAC) wrist [1]. The lateral radiograph revealed slight extension of the lunate and the presence of a humpback deformity (Fig. 10.2). Although not required, a CT scan of the wrist may provide additional information that can assist in the management of a scaphoid nonunion. It may confirm the presence of a nonunion and help quantify the amount of bone resorption and degree of humpback deformity [2, 3]. A CT scan was obtained which confirmed the absence of bone healing and the presence of a humpback deformity. An MRI without contrast is also frequently obtained to evaluate the vascularity of the proximal pole of the scaphoid [4]. This is particularly important in proximal pole fractures. If there is evidence of avascular necrosis (AVN) of the scaphoid, a vascularized bone grafting procedure is the treatment of choice. An MRI was obtained in this patient but the presence of the scaphoid screw introduced significant metallic artifact preventing adequate assessment of the vascularity of the proximal pole of the scaphoid.

Fig. 10.1 Preoperative AP X-ray demonstrating persistent scaphoid non-union. (Published with kind permission of © Roberto Diaz and James Chang, 2015. All Rights Reserved)

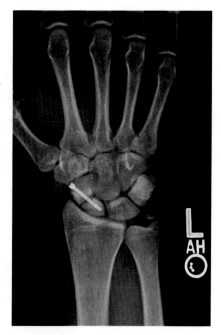

Management Options

Treatment options discussed with the patient included observation, casting, revision open reduction internal fixation with bone graft, and salvage procedures.

Management Chosen

Given the patient's persistent pain, young age, and only mild beaking of the radial styloid, revision surgical stabilization with autograft was recommended. Although the MRI could not definitively rule out proximal pole AVN due to metallic artifact, our suspicion for AVN of the proximal pole was low as the incidence of AVN is much lower following scaphoid waist fractures [5]. The

Fig. 10.2 Preoperative
lateral X-ray. (Published with
kind permission of © Roberto
Diaz and James Chang, 2015.
All Rights Reserved)

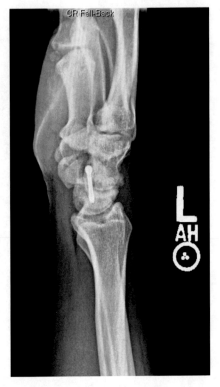

patient was consented for hardware removal, open reduction internal fixation with iliac crest bone graft (ICBG) versus vascularized
bone graft and radial styloidectomy.

Surgical Technique

Surgery was performed on an outpatient basis under general anesthesia in addition to an infraclavicular regional block for postoperative pain control. The patient was placed in the supine position with
a bump under the ipsilateral hip to facilitate ICBG harvesting. A
volar approach is preferred when correction of a humpback deformity is required. In this case, the patient's previous volar incision

Fig. 10.3 Intraoperative photograph of the volar approach. (Published with kind permission of © Roberto Diaz and James Chang, 2015. All Rights Reserved)

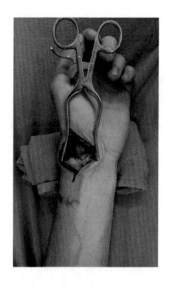

was used to access the scaphoid and the radial styloid (Fig. 10.3). A radial styloidectomy was performed and previous hardware was removed. The scaphoid fracture was identified and the presence of a nonunion was confirmed. The proximal and distal poles were excavated and all nonviable bone was removed. Bleeding was noted at the proximal pole and therefore, a vascularized bone graft was deemed unnecessary. Scaphoid length and alignment were obtained using a small lamina spreader and Kirschner wires (K-wires) as joysticks. A guidewire was then placed in the center–center position in a retrograde fashion for later placement of a headless compression screw (Fig. 10.4). Wire position was confirmed by intraoperative fluoroscopy and by visualizing the pin as it traversed the nonunion site. The appropriate screw size was then determined. A tricortical autograft wedge graft was then harvested from the ipsilateral iliac crest and contoured on the back table to the proper size. An oscillating saw was then used to create a sagittal slit in the graft to allow placement of the graft over the central scaphoid K-wire (Fig. 10.5). The graft was then inserted into the defect and a derotational K-wire was placed. A compression screw was then inserted over the central guidewire and good compression was observed

Fig. 10.4 Intraoperative
photograph illustrating exca-
vation of nonviable bone and
K-wire placement. (Publis-
hed with kind permission of
© Roberto Diaz and James
Chang, 2015. All Rights
Reserved)

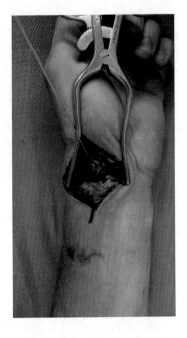

across the graft (Fig. 10.6, 10.7 and 10.8). The patient was immobilized in a sugar tong splint to prevent forearm rotation.

Clinical Course and Outcome

The patient returned to clinic 2 weeks following his surgery and
was transitioned into a short-arm thumb spica cast. A bone stimula-
tor was initiated to help promote bone healing. Serial X-rays were
obtained at 4-week intervals to evaluate progressive bone healing.
The patient was immobilized for a total of 12 weeks. Postoperative
X-rays obtained at 12 weeks are shown in Figs. 10.6–10.8. A CT
scan obtained at the 12-week mark confirmed near complete union
of the scaphoid fracture (Fig. 10.9). Physical therapy was started at
the 12-week postoperative visit. At 2 years 5 months postsurgery,
the patient was working as a greenskeeper and window washer and

Fig. 10.5 Intraoperative photograph after preparation of iliac crest bone graft and recipient site. Note the slit in the middle of the tricortical wedge to allow for insertion over the K-wire. (Published with kind permission of © Roberto Diaz and James Chang, 2015. All Rights Reserved)

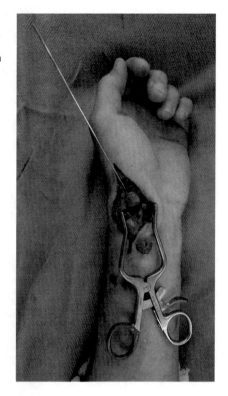

was able to perform all work duties without difficulty. Although he has not returned to competitive mountain biking, he does plan to return to this sport in the future. His patient-rated wrist evaluation total score was 6.5 and his quick disabilities of the arm, shoulder, and hand score was 2.3. Range of motion and strength in the operative and uninjured wrists were comparable as illustrated in Table 10.1.

Clinical Pearls/Pitfalls

- It is imperative that all nonviable bone be debrided from the nonunion site

Fig. 10.6 Twelve-week postoperative AP radiograph. (Published with kind permission of © Roberto Diaz and James Chang, 2015. All Rights Reserved)

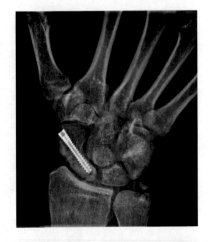

Fig. 10.7 Twelve-week postoperative oblique radiograph. (Published with kind permission of © Roberto Diaz and James Chang, 2015. All Rights Reserved)

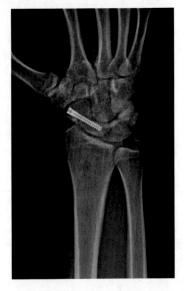

- A derotational pin is essential during placement of compression screw
- Inadequate correction of humpback deformity must be avoided and intraoperative radiographs are useful

Fig. 10.8 Twelve-week postoperative lateral radiograph. (Published with kind permission of © Roberto Diaz and James Chang, 2015. All Rights Reserved)

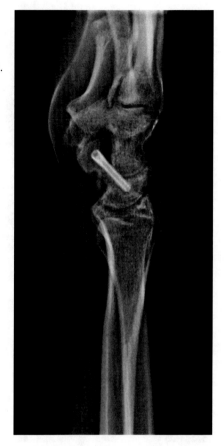

- Unrecognized avascular necrosis of the proximal pole of the scaphoid may be a pitfall and the need for a vascularized bone graft should be discussed with the patient preoperatively
- Postoperative immobilization should be continued until radiographic union is established via X-rays and/or CT scan
- Improper screw position and length of screw should be avoided and checked under fluoroscopy

Fig. 10.9 Twelve-week CT scan demonstrating healing and incorporation of the ICBG. *ICBG* iliac crest bone graft. (Published with kind permission of © Roberto Diaz and James Chang, 2015. All Rights Reserved)

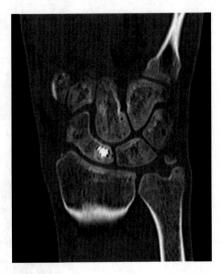

Table 10.1 Range of motion and strength at 2 years 5 months postsurgery

	Operative left wrist	Uninjured right wrist
Wrist flexion (deg)	75	85
Wrist extension (deg)	72	77
Wrist ulnar deviation (deg)	40	45
Wrist radial deviation (deg)	30	30
Grip strenth (kg)	62	60
Key pinch (kg)	8	11
Tip pinch (kg)	13	14

Literature Review and Discussion

Scaphoid waist nonunion rates have been reported in the literature as 12 % [6]. Risk factors for the development of a nonunion include delay in treatment, proximal pole fractures, fracture displacement, and inadequate immobilization [7–9]. The patient in this case was appropriately diagnosed with a scaphoid fracture and underwent a trial of nonoperative management with casting; however, he reported that he was only immobilized for 4 weeks. For acute nondisplaced scaphoid fractures treated nonoperatively, we generally recommend a period of 6–12 weeks of casting guided by radiographic evidence of healing. Inadequate immobilization may have played a role in the development of a nonunion in this case. We routinely obtain a CT scan as it can provide additional information to help guide treatment such as the degree of humpback deformity and the amount of bone resorption. A significant humpback deformity is best treated with structural bone graft through a volar approach. An MRI can assist the diagnosis of proximal pole AVN in which case a vascularized bone graft should be utilized. Treatment in the form of radial styloidectomy and ORIF with vascularized versus non-vascularized bone graft were discussed with the patient in detail. A radial styloidectomy was recommended as there were radial styloid changes consistent with an early stage I SNAC wrist and may have contributed to radial-sided pain. Intraoperatively, punctate bleeding was present at the proximal pole obviating the need for a vascularized bone graft procedure. Structural ICBG was preferred as it facilitates correction of the humpback deformity and because good healing rates have been reported in the literature. A large bone graft can also be obtained from the iliac crest that can later be contoured accordingly.

In 1960, Russe described the use of ICBG as an inlay technique and reported a 90 % union rate in 22 patients [10]. In this technique, a cavity is created in the proximal and distal poles of the scaphoid and a peg of ICBG is placed firmly within the cavities. However, correction of a humpback deformity is difficult to achieve using this technique. In 1984, Fernandez described a modification of the Fisk technique for the treatment of scaphoid nonunions associated with a humpback deformity [11, 12]. A corticocancellous ICBG is contoured into a wedge of bone that is placed into the nonunion site to restore scaphoid length and correct any angular deformity. The graft is then stabilized with K-wires. The author reported a 100 % union rate in 6 patients along with the normalization of the scapholunate angle. Filan and Herbert reported their experience using a Herbert screw in the treatment of scaphoid fractures [13]. Fractures were classified according to the Herbert classification. One hundred and seven scaphoid body-type D2 and D3 fractures were treated with corticocancellous ICBG and a Herbert screw. The union rate was 76% for type D2 fractures and 58% for type D3 fractures. In 1996, Daly et al. reported their results using a similar technique with the addition of a Herbert screw for internal fixation [14]. They achieved a 95% union rate in 26 patients with a scaphoid waist nonunion treated with a corticocancellous ICBG and a Herbert screw. Our technique is similar to that described by previous authors [12–14] but differs in that we prefer to place a guidewire prior to insertion of the corticocancellous graft. Placing a guidewire prior to graft insertion allows direct visualization of the guidewire, which ensures that it is placed along the central axis of the scaphoid. The guidewire also helps distract the proximal and distal scaphoid fragments for proper sizing of the graft and facilitate graft placement. This temporary fixation also maintains correction of the humback deformity prior to graft insertion. The disadvantage of this technique is that it requires creation of a saggital slit in the graft so that it can be placed over the guidewire as it traverses the nonunion site. This saggital slit places the graft at risk for fracture. However, fracturing the graft can be avoided through proper handling of the graft during creation of the saggital slit and during graft insertion.

Scaphoid nonunions present a challenge to both the patient and the treating physician. A thorough preoperative evaluation is particularly important in patients with persistent nonunions after prior treatment. Smoking cessation should be advocated in any patient who reports tobacco use. It is important to discuss all aspects of treatment including surgical technique, period of immobilization, rehabilitation, expected outcomes, risk of nonunion, and possible need for additional procedures.

References

1. Watson HK, Ballet FL. The SLAC wrist: scapholunate advanced collapse pattern of degenerative arthritis. J Hand Surg Am. 1984;9:358–65.
2. Amadio PC, Berquist TH, Smith DK, Illstrup DM, Cooney III WP, Linscheid RL. Scaphoid malunion. J Hand Surg Am. 1989;14:679–87.
3. Trumble TE, Salas P, Barthel T, Robert III KQ. Management of scaphoid nonunions. J Am Acad Orthop Surg. 2003;11:380–91.
4. Trumble TE: Avascular necrosis after scaphoid fracture: a correlation of magnetic resonance imaging and histology. J Hand Surg Am. 1990;15:557–64.
5. Gelberman RH, Menon J. The vascularity of the scaphoid bone. J Hand Surg Am. 1980;5:508–13.
6. Dias JJ, Brenkel IJ, Finlay DB. Patterns of union in fractures of the waist of the scaphoid. J Bone Joint Surg Br. 1989;71:307–10.
7. Kawamura K, Chung KC. Treatment of scaphoid fractures and nonunions. J Hand Surg Am. 2008;33(6):988–97.
8. Buijze GA, Ochtma L, Ring D. Management of scaphoid nonunion. J Hand Surg Am. 2012;37:1095–100.
9. Wong K, Von Scroeder H. Delays and poor management of scaphoid fractures contributing to nonunion. J Hand Surg Am. 2011;36(9):1471–4.
10. Russe O. Fracture of the carpal navicular: diagnosis, non-operative treatment and operative treatment. J Bone Joint Surg Am. 1960; 42:759–68.
11. Fisk GR. Operative surgery, part II. In: Bentley G, editor. Orthopaedics. Kent: Butterworths; 1979. p 540.
12. Fernandez DL. A technique for anterior wedge-shaped grafts for scaphoid nonunions with carpal instability. J Hand Surg Am. 1984;9:733–7.
13. Filan SL, Herbert TJ. Herbert screw fixation of scaphoid fractures. J Bone Joint Surg Br. 1996;78:519–29.
14. Daly K, Gill P, Magnussen PA, Simonis RB. Established nonunion of the scaphoid treated by volar wedge grafting and Herbert screw fixation. J Bone Joint Surg Br. 1996;78(4):530–4.

Chapter 11
The Hybrid Russe Graft for the Treatment of Scaphoid Nonunion

Steve K. Lee and Scott W. Wolfe

Case Presentation

The patient was a 25-year-old right hand dominant male professional basketball player with the chief complaint of right wrist pain. He had sustained a fall while playing basketball 9 months prior to presentation. He had radiographs by an outside physician and was told they were negative. He continued to have pain and was unable to play. He was otherwise healthy and took no medications.

Physical Assessment

The scaphoid was tender to palpation at the anatomic snuffbox. Wrist flexion was 60° and extension was 55°. There was a negative Watson scaphoid shift test. The patient had full digital range of motion and was neurovascularly intact distally.

S. K. Lee (✉) ·S. W. Wolfe
Department of Orthopaedic Surgery, Hospital for Special Surgery, Weill Medical College of Cornell University, New York, NY, USA
e-mail: steve.kichul.lee@gmail.com; lees@hss.edu

S. W. Wolfe
Professor of Orthopaedic Surgery, Hospital for Special Surgery, Weill Medical College of Cornell University, New York, NY, USA
e-mail: wolfes@hss.edu

© Springer International Publishing Switzerland 2015
J. Yao (ed.), *Scaphoid Fractures and Nonunions,*
DOI 10.1007/978-3-319-18977-2_11

Diagnostic Studies

Plain radiographs (Figs. 11.1, 11.2) and CT scan showed a scaphoid waist nonunion with a flexion humpback deformity (Fig. 11.3) of the scaphoid and dorsal intercalated segmental instability (DISI) pattern of the carpus. There was no obvious evidence of vascular compromise.

Diagnosis

Scaphoid waist nonunion with humpback deformity and DISI.

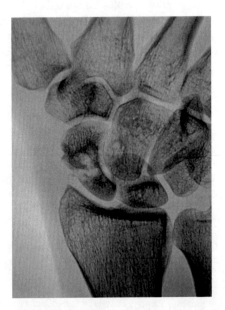

Fig. 11.1 Scaphoid nonunion, preoperative radiograph, wrist PA view. *PA* posterior-anterior. (Published with kind permission of © Steve K. Lee 2015. All Rights Reserved)

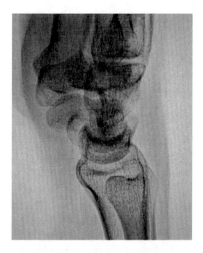

Fig. 11.2 Scaphoid nonunion, preoperative radiograph, wrist lateral view. (Published with kind permission of © Steve K. Lee 2015. All Rights Reserved)

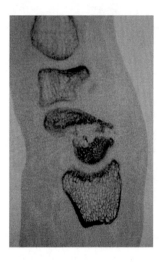

Fig. 11.3 Scaphoid nonunion, preoperative CT scan, sagittal view with humpback deformity. (Published with kind permission of © Steve K. Lee 2015. All Rights Reserved)

Management Options

Nonoperative treatment (immobilization, bone stimulation) could be employed but has a very low likelihood of gaining union in this chronic, displaced scaphoid fracture with deformity. Further delay in treatment may lead to scaphoid nonunion advanced collapse (SNAC) [1–3]. Surgical options included reduction, bone grafting, internal fixation, and autogenous nonvascularized or vascularized graft [4]. The usual donor site choices for nonvascularized autograft include the distal radius, iliac crest, proximal ulna, and proximal tibia [4]. Vascularized bone graft choices include a local pedicled type such as the 1,2 intercompartmental supraretinacular artery radial bone graft [5, 6], the first dorsal intermetacarpal artery graft [7], the Mathoulin volar pedicle graft [8, 9], and free vascularized tissue transfer such as from the medial femoral condyle [10, 11].

Management Chosen

Our preference for treatment in these scenarios is the hybrid Russe autograft technique. It employs a nonvascularized distal radius cortical strut and cancellous autograft, combined with a headless compression screw (Fig. 11.4).

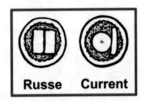

Fig. 11.4 Drawing showing axial cut through the scaphoid comparing the Russe procedure (*left*) and the current procedure (*right*) showing the position of the screw as well as the graft. In the hybrid Russe procedure, there is a much higher ratio of cancellous to cortical bone within the scaphoid. (Published with kind permission of © Steve K. Lee 2015. All Rights Reserved)

Surgical Technique

A typical hockey-stick incision is made along the course of the flexor carpi radialis (FCR) tendon and extended distally along the border of the glabrous skin of the thenar eminence to the STT joint. Splitting the sheath of the FCR allows the FCR to be retracted ulnarly. The floor of the FCR sheath is incised longitudinally to expose the wrist capsule and extrinsic ligaments. The superficial branch of the radial artery to the superficial arch is typically divided between sutures. The distal and proximal poles of the scaphoid are exposed with a capsular incision in line with the scaphoid axis, and the extrinsic capsular ligaments are carefully tagged with nonabsorbable suture for later repair. The wrist is extended over a rolled towel, and the nonunion is gapped open using skin hooks in the proximal and distal fragments (Fig. 11.5).

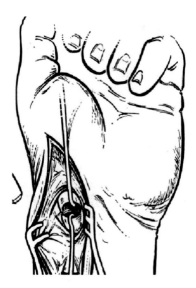

Fig. 11.5 Standard Russe incision between the FCR and radial artery. Nonunion site is exposed with the aid of skin hooks. Fibrous tissue resected. The scaphoid poles are curetted to concave, bleeding surfaces proximally and distally. *FCR* flexor carpi radialis. (Published with kind permission of © Steve K. Lee, 2015. All Rights Reserved)

All fibrous tissue at the nonunion site is removed and bone is curretted to remove sclerotic bone and fibrous tissue down to bleeding cancellous bone. The prepared cavity is measured to judge the size of the cortical strut, which is generally 12–18 mm.

In cases of humpback deformity and DISI, the lunate must be reduced. This may be done with a wrist flexion maneuver to reduce the extended lunate and proximal scaphoid pole, followed by the placement of a percutaneous radiolunate 0.062 in K-wire. The wire may be placed from a dorsal or a radial insertion site across the radius and into the reduced lunate. The wire is either buried below the skin or left out of the skin depending on surgeon preference, and left in place for 4 weeks, providing additional stability to the scaphoid construct. The wrist is then extended to reduce the distal scaphoid pole and restore alignment.

After preparation and cavitation of the scaphoid, proximal dissection is performed to expose the bone graft site in the metaphysis of the radius. The pronator quadratus is reflected ulnarwards off the radial metaphysis. A 20 × 5 mm rounded cortical window is then made from the volar cortex of the distal radius using osteotomes or K-wires, and the cortical fragment is set aside for later use (Fig. 11.6). Abundant cancellous bone graft is harvested from the radius. A "matchstick" is fabricated from the volar cortical window of the radius and sized to act as an intramedullary cortical strut to restore the length and alignment of the scaphoid (Figs. 11.7, 11.8). Using bone hooks to extend the prepared proximal and distal poles, the cortical strut is inserted into the defect and tamped into position. Cancellous bone graft is then packed tightly in the remainder of the nonunion site, and this is followed with fixation with a headless scaphoid screw (Figs. 11.9, 11.10), generally inserted from distal to proximal. Intraoperative fluoroscopy is used to confirm adequate reduction and fixation. The volar capsule and radiocarpal ligaments are repaired with interrupted nonabsorbable sutures. In the case of previous surgery, this technique may still be used, but the new and/or larger diameter screw should be placed in a different track if technically feasible. The cortical strut may be inserted down the previous screw tract. Also, if there is difficulty getting the screw guidewire in the optimal position in the scaphoid from the volar approach, a mini incision is made dorsally and the screw is placed from the dorsal approach.

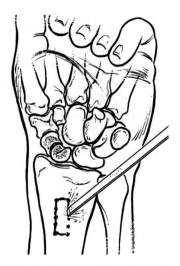

Fig. 11.6 A cortical window (20 × 5 mm) is made on the volar cortex of the distal radius. It is imperative that this cortical piece is harvested intact without fracture. Cancellous bone graft is harvested from the metaphyseal distal radius. (Published with kind permission of © Steve K. Lee 2015. All Rights Reserved)

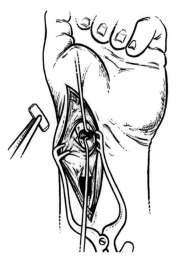

Fig. 11.7 A "matchstick" that is made from the volar cortex of the distal radius is sculpted to the appropriate size. The scaphoid poles are hyperextended and the matchstick is placed *inside* the nonunion site as a strut. (Published with kind permission of © Steve K. Lee 2015. All Rights Reserved)

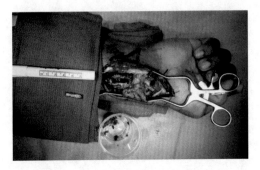

Fig. 11.8 Intraoperative view of bone graft harvest from volar distal radius. (Published with kind permission of © Steve K. Lee 2015. All Rights Reserved)

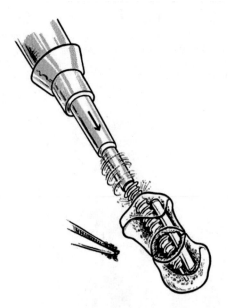

Fig. 11.9 Cancellous bone graft is packed in the remainder of the non-union site, followed by fixation with a headless compression screw. Note the matchstick strut is *within* the scaphoid, not wedged on the volar cortical surface. (Published with kind permission of © Steve K. Lee 2015. All Rights Reserved)

Postoperatively, the patient is initially splinted for 2 weeks. For patients with a radiolunate wire, above elbow immobilization for 4 weeks is recommended to prevent wire breakage. The wire is removed at 4 weeks, and a short-arm thumb spica cast is applied until healing. A CT scan is performed to confirm union at 10–14 weeks postoperatively, and immobilization is converted to a custom-molded removable splint until comfortable.

Clinical Course and Outcome

The patient underwent the hybrid Russe technique as described above and healed at 12 weeks (Figs. 11.11, 11.12), as confirmed with CT scan (Figs. 11.13, 11.14). At 5 months postoperatively, the patient demonstrated wrist flexion of 70°, extension of 60°,

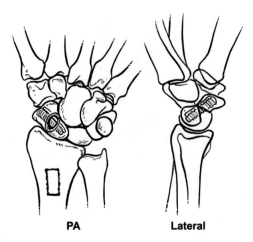

PA   **Lateral**

Fig. 11.10 PA and lateral drawings showing the scaphoid after hybrid Russe procedure. The humpback deformity has been corrected and the length of the scaphoid has been restored. A headless compression screw provides additional fixation to the construct. *PA* posterior-anterior. (Published with kind permission of © Steve K. Lee 2015. All Rights Reserved)

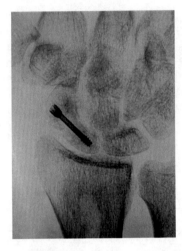

Fig. 11.11 Postoperative radiograph, wrist PA view. *PA* posterior-anterior. (Published with kind permission of © Steve K. Lee 2015. All Rights Reserved)

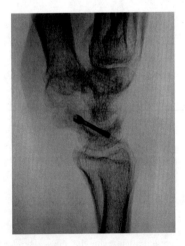

Fig. 11.12 Postoperative radiograph, wrist lateral view. (Published with kind permission of © Steve K. Lee 2015. All Rights Reserved)

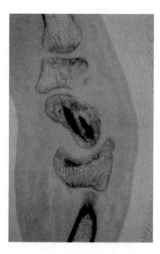

Fig. 11.13 Postoperative CT scan, sagittal view, revealing the healed scaphoid. Note the dense cortical bone strut within the scaphoid. (Published with kind permission of © Steve K. Lee 2015. All Rights Reserved)

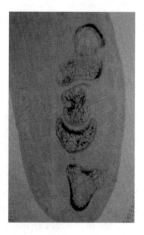

Fig. 11.14 Postoperative CT scan, sagittal view, revealing the corrected DISI. *DISI* dorsal intercalated segmental instability. (Published with kind permission of © Steve K. Lee 2015. All Rights Reserved)

radial and ulnar deviation of 10 and 40°, respectively, and supination/pronation of 80 and 85°. Grip strength was 100 pounds versus 110 on the contralateral side. Pinch strength was 20 pounds bilaterally. He returned to play professional basketball.

Clinical Pearls/Pitfalls

Keys to attain healing are as follows:

- Good preparation of the donor site to cancellous bone
- Correction of DISI alignment and placement of a temporary 0.062" radiolunate K-wire as necessary
- Placement of the cortical intramedullary strut to reconstruct intrascaphoid angle and carpal alignment
- High cancellous to cortical bone ratio with tight packing in the fracture site
- Stable fixation with an intramedullary screw
- In patients with a small proximal pole or tenuous fixation, an additional 0.062" K-wire from the distal scaphoid to the capitate will neutralize the long moment arm and increase construct stability
- Indications are scaphoid waist or proximal pole nonunion
- Ischemia is not a contraindication

Literature Review and Discussion

Scaphoid nonunions continue to be a challenging problem for which the ideal treatment remains controversial. We introduce the hybrid Russe procedure as a straightforward method to reduce the deformity, attain rigid fixation, and provide abundant bone graft to stimulate healing. Green described Otto Russe's visit to San Antonio in his landmark paper [12, 13]. Green's modified Russe technique was one where there were back-to-back corticocancellous struts from the iliac crest placed in an intramedullary fashion, surrounded by cancellous graft. No fixation was used. We modified this technique to combine the advantages of this classic technique with the rigid fixation of a headless screw, and call it the "hybrid Russe" technique. The cortical strut of the radial volar cortex is substantially thinner than the iliac crest and allows packing with a higher volume of cancellous bone.

In a retrospective review of our series of hybrid Russe for scaphoid waist and proximal pole nonunions, 17 male and 3 female patients (mean age 31), with a mean follow-up period of 28.9 months, were examined clinically and with radiographs. No patients were excluded secondary to ischemia. All 20 scaphoids healed and the mean time for healing was 3.4 months. The mean postoperative intrascaphoid angle was significantly reduced, from 63.9° preoperatively to 35.6° postoperatively. Similarly, the mean radiolunate angle was significantly improved from $-18.4°$ preoperatively to $-1.2°$ postoperatively. The scapholunate angle also demonstrated significant improvement from 68.8° preoperatively to 52.8° postoperatively. Grip strength improved from 78.9% of contralateral hand to 90.9% following the procedure. All patients were satisfied with the functional outcome upon follow-up, and no site morbidity, or hardware, issues were reported [14]. This procedure is indicated for waist and proximal pole nonunions, irregardless of vascularity. We have been successful getting both types to heal. We are now embarking on a scaphoid pathology (from the nonunion site) versus MRI versus healing study.

A modification of the Russe technique using the volar cortex of the distal radius as a cortical strut, followed by packing of cancellous bone and headless screw fixation for the treatment of scaphoid nonunions, is a method with encouraging early results. This method restores and maintains the carpal alignment, while avoiding the donor site morbidities associated with iliac crest bone graft harvesting. This technique provides excellent radiographic and functional results. We recommend this technique to treat scaphoid waist nonunions.

Acknowledgment The authors would like to thank Zina Model, BA, for her editorial assistance.

References

1. Mack GR, Bosse MJ, Gelberman RH, Yu E. The natural history of scaphoid non-union. J Bone Joint Surg Am. 1984;66(4):504–9.
2. Vender MI, Watson HK, Wiener BD, Black DM. Degenerative change in symptomatic scaphoid nonunion. J Hand Surg Am. 1987;12(4):514–9.
3. Ruby LK, Cooney WP, 3rd, An KN, Linscheid RL, Chao EY. Relative motion of selected carpal bones: a kinematic analysis of the normal wrist. J Hand Surg Am. 1988;13(1):1–10.
4. Stark A, Brostrom LA, Svartengren G. Surgical treatment of scaphoid nonunion. Review of the literature and recommendations for treatment. Arch Orthop Trauma Surg. 1989;108(4):203–9.
5. Zaidemberg C, Siebert JW, Angrigiani C. A new vascularized bone graft for scaphoid nonunion. J Hand Surg Am. 1991;16(3):474–8.
6. Steinmann SP, Bishop AT, Berger RA. Use of the 1,2 intercompartmental supraretinacular artery as a vascularized pedicle bone graft for difficult scaphoid nonunion. J Hand Surg Am. 2002;27(3):391–401.
7. Fernandez DL, Eggli S. Non-union of the scaphoid. Revascularization of the proximal pole with implantation of a vascular bundle and bone-grafting. J Bone Joint Surg Am. 1995;77(6):883–93.
8. Mathoulin C, Brunelli F. Further experience with the index metacarpal vascularized bone graft. J Hand Surg Br. 1998;23(3):311–7.
9. Mathoulin C, Haerle M. Vascularized bone graft from the palmar carpal artery for treatment of scaphoid nonunion. J Hand Surg Br. 1998;23(3):318–23.
10. Jones DB, Jr, Moran SL, Bishop AT, Shin AY. Free-vascularized medial femoral condyle bone transfer in the treatment of scaphoid nonunions. Plast Reconstr Surg. 2010;125(4):1176–84.
11. Yamamoto H, Jones DB, Jr, Moran SL, Bishop AT, Shin AY. The arterial anatomy of the medial femoral condyle and its clinical implications. J Hand Surg Eur Vol. 2010;35(7):569–74.
12. Green DP. The effect of avascular necrosis on Russe bone grafting for scaphoid nonunion. J Hand Surg Am. 1985;10(5):597–605.
13. RUSSE O. Fracture of the carpal navicular. Diagnosis, non-operative treatment, and operative treatment. J Bone Joint Surg Am. 1960;42-A:759–68.
14. Roman J, Lockyer P, Paksima N, Lee S. The modified russe procedure for scaphoid waist fracture non-union with deformity. Feb 7, 2012.

Chapter 12
Arthroscopic Grafting and Scapholunate Pinning for Scaphoid Proximal Pole Nonunion

Christophe Mathoulin

Case Presentation

An otherwise healthy 23-year-old metalworker, without any previous medical history other than smoking, was presented in March 2010 after falling on his left wrist during a motorcycle accident. His wrist had been immobilized in a splint without X-rays being taken. Pain had disappeared during the third week, so the splint was removed and he started using his hand normally. One year later, the pain recurred and then increased. He consulted his doctor who found a proximal pole fracture with a very small proximal fragment of the scaphoid on X-rays. The patient was sent to a specialized surgical center 18 months after the initial injury.

Physical Assessment

- Pain score was 7 on the VAS scale
- Extension was 60 vs. 85° on the opposite side
- Flexion was 60 vs. 80° on the opposite side
- Radial deviation was 10 vs. 30° on the opposite side

C. Mathoulin (✉)
Institut de la Main, Hand department, Clinique Jouvenet, Paris, France
e-mail: cmathoulin@orange.fr

© Springer International Publishing Switzerland 2015   137
J. Yao (ed.), *Scaphoid Fractures and Nonunions,*
DOI 10.1007/978-3-319-18977-2_12

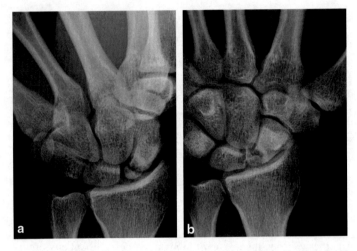

Fig. 12.1 a–b X-rays of very small proximal pole nonunion. (Published with kind permission of ©Christophe Mathoulin 2015. All Rights Reserved)

- Ulnar deviation was 20 vs. 40° on the opposite side
- Full pronation and supination
- Grip strength was 30 kg versus 50 kg on the opposite side
- Disabilities of arm, shoulder and hand (DASH) score was 80.82

Diagnostic Studies

- X-rays showed a very proximal nonunion of the scaphoid's proximal pole with bone loss. There were no signs of necrosis (Fig. 12.1a, b).

Management Options

Conventional grafting by open techniques does not always achieve a satisfactory union rate. The advent of vascularized grafts was an indisputable technical advancement that enhanced the vascularity of the proximal pole and improved the union rate. However, the surgical technique is challenging, especially in the case of a small proximal pole fragment.

Management Chosen

After a discussion with the patient, he agreed to completely stop smoking for a minimum of 1 month before surgery. The surgical procedure consisted of a fixation method that captured the body and proximal pole of the scaphoid, along with the lunate in the radio-ulnar axis, in combination with insertion of cancellous bone autograft.

Surgical Procedure

The patient was operated 1 month and a half after smoking cessation. The procedure was performed on an outpatient basis under regional anesthesia and with an arm tourniquet.

First Step: Graft Harvesting The graft was harvested from the lateral radius through a longitudinal incision centered over the radial styloid process. The cutaneous and sensory branches of the radial nerve were protected. Subperiosteal dissection between the first and second extensor compartments was carried out to keep the tendon sheaths intact. A three-sided osteotomy was made on the lateral cortex of the radial styloid; a bone lid was created that had a proximal hinge. The graft was harvested with a curette and about twice the estimated volume of the defect was taken. The bone lid was then repositioned and the first and second compartments were spontaneously repositioned so as to stabilize the harvest site.

Second Step: Arthroscopic Bone Grafting Axial traction was placed on the wrist. The arthroscope was inserted into the midcarpal joint through the ulnar midcarpal portal (2 cm distal and 2 cm ulnar to Lister's tubercle) to explore the distal aspect of the scaphoid. The nonunion was confirmed. Reduction was achieved using simple axial traction on the thumb. Thorough cleaning and

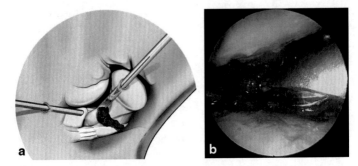

Fig. 12.2 **a** Drawing and **b** arthroscopic view showing the way to push the cancellous bone graft into the bone loss of the scaphoid nonunion, using the burr. (Published with kind permission of ©Christophe Mathoulin 2015. All Rights Reserved)

curettage of the two scaphoid surfaces was carried out using a curette and shaver through the radial midcarpal portal (2 cm distal to Lister's tubercle). This step can be done with or without fluid; however, dry arthroscopy is required for graft insertion. The cannula from a 3.0-mm burr was inserted through the radial midcarpal portal up to the defect between the proximal pole and the body of the scaphoid. The graft material was pushed using the head of the burr into the bone defect site, and then compacted using a spatula (Figs. 12.2a, b).

Third Step: Fixation by Scapholunate Pinning We used a typical percutaneous scapholunate pinning method under arthroscopic and fluoroscopic control. Two pins were driven percutaneously into the radial aspect of the wrist, through the distal body of the scaphoid, so as to bridge the graft area, secure the proximal pole and then was advanced into the lunate (Fig. 12.3).

The arthroscopic portal incisions were not closed. A simple volar splint in slight wrist extension was used by the patient until bone union was achieved. X-rays were taken every 15 days. The pins were removed in the second month after union. Rehabilitation was started immediately thereafter (Figs. 12.4a, b, c).

Fig. 12.3 Postoperative X-rays showing the special trick of scapholunate pinning. (Published with kind permission of ©Christophe Mathoulin 2015. All Rights Reserved)

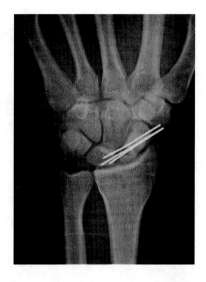

Clinical Course and Outcome

At final follow-up in the 30th month, the patient had obtained union, and the pain had disappeared completely and the VAS was 0 (Figs. 12.5a, b, c). The DASH was 0 with no functional impairment.

Extension was 80°, flexion was 80°, radial deviation was 25°, ulnar deviation was 40°, and pronation and supination were possible over the full range of motion and grip strength was 55 kg. Figure 12.6 demonstrates the clinical view of the final result with complete range of motion.

Clinical Pearls/Pitfalls

- Arthroscopic technique requires only a local-regional anesthesia
- First step is to harvest the cancellous bone graft from distal radius by lateral 1–2 approach, keeping the cortical bone to close the graft donor area

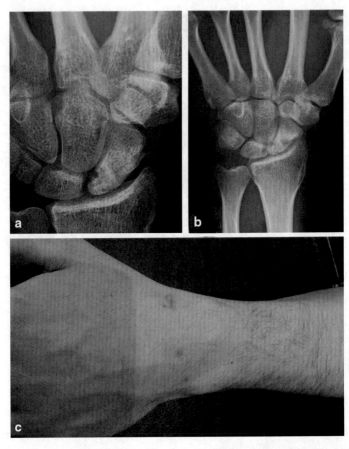

Fig. 12.4 a, b, c X-rays and clinical view of wrist at 45 days after the removal of K-wires. (Published with kind permission of ©Christophe Mathoulin 2015. All Rights Reserved)

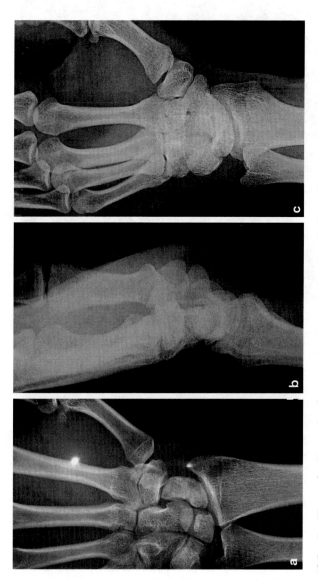

Fig. 12.5 a, b, c X-rays after 2 years showing a complete reconstruction of scaphoid. (Published with kind permission of ©Christophe Mathoulin 2015. All Rights Reserved)

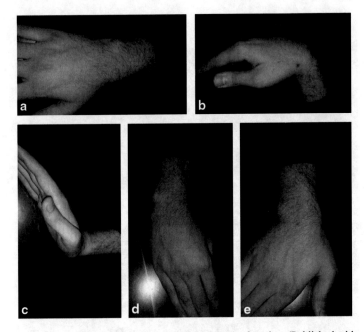

Fig. 12.6 a–e The final result with complete range of motion. (Published with kind permission of ©Christophe Mathoulin 2015. All Rights Reserved)

- Midcarpal portals are classically sufficient to check and treat the nonunion area. Ulnar midcarpal portal for scope and radial midcarpal portal for grafting
- Implementation of the graft should be done without water in the procedure of dry arthroscopy
- No need to fix the cancellous bone graft, the shape of capitate maintain bone graft in a good position after releasing tension
- The fixation of scaphoid needs a lateral scapholunate pinning, fixing distal scaphoid, graft area, proximal pole, and lunate

Literature Review and Discussion

The treatment of scaphoid nonunion has long been controversial and different techniques have been described. Fractures of the proximal pole are susceptible to nonunion because of its precarious blood supply. The small size of the proximal fragment makes it less amenable to standard fixation techniques and leads to divergent results.

Ho has shown arthroscopic bone grafting to be an effective treatment of scaphoid nonunion; preservation of the scaphoid's vascularity was an asset [1]. At the proximal pole, especially in small fragments, not opening or touching the structures that provide blood to the proximal pole (scapholunate ligament, dorsal and volar extrinsic wrist ligaments) is a key point in this technique. Graft insertion is easily done arthroscopically. Ho recommends using biological glue to stabilize the cancellous graft once implanted. In our experience, this is not necessary—when traction is released, the anatomical position of the capitate fits into the curvature of the scaphoid and stabilizes the graft material.

Ho also recommends harvesting grafts from the iliac crest. We have always preferred harvesting bone from the radius for two reasons: The patient is usually young and the quality of the cancellous bone of the radius is excellent. As a consequence, the procedure can be performed as an outpatient procedure under regional anesthesia, which is very popular with patients.

Fixation is no longer done with conventional retrograde screws, which are not a good indication in this proximal location, or with anterograde screws given the small size of the fragment. Placing a proximal screw in such a small fragment induces a significant risk of fracture, along with the fact that is passes through an important area of the cartilage in the radiocarpal joint.

We chose to perform an original, more anatomical scapholunate pinning method, which provides excellent stabilization of the graft and the proximal pole. Fixation between the scaphoid and lunate is very easy to achieve. The pins are cut under the skin and removed after union. In our first series, the union rate was 100% with an average time of 8 weeks (unpublished data). In a more recent series involving only the proximal pole, the union rate was excellent, with only one case of delayed union at 6 months (unpublished data).

Another important point to consider is that smoking must be stopped completely, at least until union is achieved. In our experience, smokers have a much lower union rate than nonsmokers. This pretext must be used to help patients stop smoking, which was achieved in all cases in our series.

Arthroscopic bone grafting associated with an original scapholunate pinning method for treating proximal pole nonunion of the scaphoid is an elegant and simple technique that is less traumatic for the patient and results in an excellent union rate.

Reference

1. Ho PC, Hung LK. Arthroscopic bone grafting in scaphoid nonunion and delayed union. In: Slutsky D, Slade J, editors. The scaphoid. NY: Thieme; 2001. pp. 131–43.

Chapter 13
1,2 ICSRA for the Management of Proximal Pole Scaphoid Nonunion

Harvey Chim, David G. Dennison and Sanjeev Kakar

Case Presentation

A 24-year-old woman injured her right wrist in a car accident 6 months prior to presentation. She did not initially seek medical attention for the wrist injury. However, she had persistent right wrist pain, and subsequently sought medical attention 6 months after the initial injury. Her pain was worse with grip and exertion, but she was otherwise able to use her wrist for other activities of daily living. Her past medical history was unremarkable.

Physical Assessment

Musculoskeletal examination revealed relatively well-preserved wrist motion, with wrist extension of 70° and flexion of 100° on the right, as opposed to wrist extension of 85° on the right and

S. Kakar (✉) · D. G. Dennison
Department of Orthopaedic Surgery, Mayo Clinic, 200 1st Street SW, Rochester, MN 55905, USA
e-mail: kakar.sanjeev@mayo.edu

H. Chim
Department of Orthopaedics, Mayo Clinic, 200 1st Street SW, Rochester, MN 55905, USA
e-mail: Chim.Harvey@mayo.edu

© Springer International Publishing Switzerland 2015   147
J. Yao (ed.), *Scaphoid Fractures and Nonunions,*
DOI 10.1007/978-3-319-18977-2_13

flexion of 105° on the left (normal) side. Ulnar deviation was 55° on the right and radial deviation was 20° on the right, as opposed to ulnar deviation of 60° and radial deviation of 30° on the left side. Grip strength on the right was 36 kg, while that on the left was 30 kg. Appositional pinch was 6.5 kg on the right and 6 kg on the left. On the right wrist, Watson's test was negative and she had point tenderness over the proximal scaphoid which reproduced her daily symptoms of pain.

Diagnostic Studies

Plain radiographs of the right wrist revealed a proximal pole nonunion of the scaphoid at the level of the proximal pole, without humpback deformity. This was confirmed on CT of the right wrist (Fig. 13.1) that showed the nonunion with minimal extension of the lunate. An MRI was obtained and was concerning for avascular necrosis (AVN) of the proximal pole.

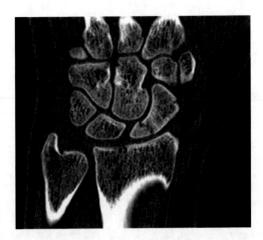

Fig. 13.1 Preoperative CT scan shows nonunion of a scaphoid proximal pole fracture. (Published with kind permission of ©Harvey Chim, David G. Dennison, and Sanjeev Kakar, 2015. All Rights Reserved)

Diagnosis

The patient was diagnosed with a nonunited proximal pole fracture of the right scaphoid.

Management Chosen

Due to the presumed poor vascularity of the proximal pole of the scaphoid, together with the lack of a humpback deformity or lunate extension, she was considered to be a good candidate for a 1,2 intercompartmental supraretinacular artery (ICSRA) vascularized bone graft procedure. The ultimate decision about the vascularity of the proximal pole and the need for a vascularized bone graft, however, would be determined intraoperatively.

Surgical Technique

A curvilinear incision, paralleling the course of the extensor pollicis longus (EPL), was outlined over the dorsal radial border of the wrist. Gravity exsanguination was used as opposed to an Esmarch bandage to permit 1,2 ICSRA vessel identification. The superficial branches of the radial nerve were identified and protected. The 1,2 ICSRA was identified running along the extensor retinaculum between the 1st and 2nd extensor compartments. It arises from the radial artery approximately 5 cm proximal to the radiocarpal joint and passes beneath the brachioradialis to lie on the dorsal surface of the extensor retinaculum. Distally, the vessels anastomose with the radial artery within the anatomical snuffbox. It is off this distal anastomosis that this reverse-flow vascularized bone graft is based.

The transverse proximal limb of a ligament sparing capsulotomy was then made over the radiocarpal joint to expose the proximal pole of the scaphoid. The fracture site was debrided with curettes and small osteotomes to minimize any thermal necrosis that may be caused by a high-speed burr and the tourniquet deflated to examine the vascularity of the proximal pole. There was scant bleeding from the proximal pole and so a decision was made to stabilize the nonunion and augment this with the 1,2 ICSRA-fed autograft. A partially threaded cannulated headless compression screw was then passed from proximal to distal, preferentially placing the screw volarly to allow the graft to be placed dorsally. Osteotomes were then used to make a box cut dorsally around the site of the scaphoid nonunion to create a space for the vascularized bone graft (Fig. 13.2).

Attention was then turned to harvesting the bone graft. The 1,2 ICSRA vessel was identified, and the 1st and 2nd extensor compartments were opened radially and ulnarly, respectively, to leave a cuff of tissue around the pedicle of the graft. The vascularized bone graft was centered approximately 15 mm proximal to the joint line to include the nutrient vessels (Fig. 13.3). To achieve this, the proximal vessels leading to the graft were ligated. The distal pedicle was then raised off the extensor retinaculum with care to preserve their integrity as they supply the outlined graft. The graft was elevated using osteotomes, and care was taken to ensure it was not kinked or rotated as it was transposed distally.

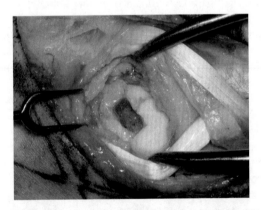

Fig. 13.2 A box cut is made around the fracture site in the scaphoid to create space for the 1,2 ICSRA vascularized bone graft. *ICSRA* intercompartmental supraretinacular artery. (Published with kind permission of ©Harvey Chim, David G. Dennison, and Sanjeev Kakar, 2015. All Rights Reserved.)

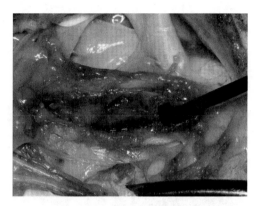

Fig. 13.3   The 1,2 ICSRA vascularized bone graft has been raised and is isolated on its pedicle. *ICSRA* intercompartmental supraretinacular artery. (Published with kind permission of ©Harvey Chim, David G. Dennison, and Sanjeev Kakar, 2015. All Rights Reserved)

A small additional wedge cut parallel to one longitudinal border of the graft can help with completing the deep cancellous cut without breaking the graft. With the tourniquet deflated, one can observe pulsatile bleeding from the bone surface. The pedicle and vascularized bone graft were then transposed distally underneath the second compartment tendons. A small amount of cancellous bone graft from the distal radius donor site was first packed into the defect, and then, the 1,2 ICSRA graft was gently tamped and pushed into place dorsally. The distal radius donor site was then packed with bone allograft and the incision closed in layers. A long-arm thumb spica splint was placed.

Clinical Course and Outcome

The patient was immobilized in a long-arm thumb spica cast for 4 weeks postoperatively and then transferred into a short-arm thumb spica cast until union. Given the difficulty associated with determination of osseous union with plain radiographs, and the prolonged average time to union with proximal pole fractures

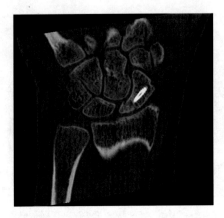

Fig. 13.4 Three-month postoperative CT scan shows union across the scaphoid proximal pole nonunion site. (Published with kind permission of ©Harvey Chim, David G. Dennison, and Sanjeev Kakar, 2015. All Rights Reserved)

[1–4], a CT scan is obtained at 12 weeks. This showed healing across the fracture site (Fig. 13.4). The patient was then placed into a thumb spica splint and gradually weaned out of this as she advanced her range of motion and strengthening exercises. At 1-year follow-up (Fig. 13.5), she had regained 75 % and 86 % of wrist extension and flexion compared to the contralateral side. Ulnar and radial deviation, as well as grip strength, were symmetrical.

Clinical Pearls/Pitfalls

- The 1,2 ICSRA pedicle should be identified prior to incising the extensor retinaculum.
- It is indicated in scaphoid proximal pole avascular nonunions without evidence of humpback deformity.
- A volarly based screw in the scaphoid allows stable fixation of the scaphoid, while allowing space for placement of the dorsal 1,2 ICSRA vascularized bone graft.

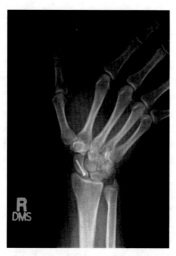

Fig. 13.5 Radiograph at 1-year postreconstruction showing union of the fractured proximal pole. (Published with kind permission of ©Harvey Chim, David G. Dennison, and Sanjeev Kakar, 2015. All Rights Reserved)

- In the presence of AVN of the proximal pole with carpal collapse, a free vascularized bone graft such as a medial femoral condyle or rib autograft may be considered as an option for treatment of the nonunited scaphoid fracture.

Literature Review and Discussion

Within the carpus, the scaphoid is the most commonly fractured, and accounts for more than 60 % of all carpal bone fractures [5]. Nonunion is a problem that is encountered particularly often with scaphoid fractures, especially in those involving the proximal one third of the scaphoid. This relates to the blood supply of the scaphoid, which is primarily derived from branches from the radial artery entering the scaphoid through foramina on its distal dorsal ridge. The vascular supply of the proximal pole hence is derived in a retrograde fashion from these vessels proceeding from distal to proximal, and is easily disrupted following a fracture. With disruption of the blood supply of the proximal pole, AVN develops in approximately 3 % of all scaphoid fractures [1]. When a scaphoid nonunion is left untreated, a predictable pattern of degenerative arthritis develops, termed scaphoid nonunion advanced collapse (SNAC), progressing from localized to pancarpal arthritis.

Various techniques have been attempted for treatment of scaphoid nonunion of the proximal pole, such as nonvascularized autografts from the iliac crest or internal fixation with a screw alone. However, these techniques have had limited success, due to the poor vascularity of the proximal scaphoid pole. Vascularized pedicled bone grafts are useful in the treatment of scaphoid nonunion, and were initially reported by Zaidemberg et al. [6] for the treatment of long-standing scaphoid nonunions. Most commonly, these are based off vessels supplying the dorsal distal radius, arising from the radial artery and running in a retrograde fashion. Two consistent intercompartmental vessels exist, lying superficial to the extensor retinaculum. These are the 1,2 ICSRA and 2,3 ICSRA. Two other deep vessels arise from the dorsal carpal arch, the 4th and 5th extensor compartment arteries (ECA). The 1,2 ICSRA and 2,3 ICSRA are useful for grafting the scaphoid, while the 4th ECA is more useful for grafting the lunate due to the ulnar location of this vessel.

The 1,2 ICSRA is the most common pedicle used for vascularized bone grafts in scaphoid nonunions. It arises from the radial artery approximately 5 cm proximal to the radiocarpal joint and passes beneath the brachioradialis to lie on the dorsal surface of the extensor retinaculum. Although the pedicle has a short arc of rotation, its radial location makes it ideal for grafts to the scaphoid.

The 1,2 ICSRA vascularized bone graft has been shown to have excellent results, with union in 95 to 100 % of the patients [2, 6–9], in the absence of avascular necrosis (AVN) of the proximal pole. Despite the improvements in MRI technology, the sensitivity and specificity for the diagnosis of AVN have been quoted as 76 and 99 %, respectively, in one study [3]. Given this, the most accurate determination of avascularity is the absence of punctate bleeding noted intraoperatively with the tourniquet deflated [4, 8]. With AVN of the proximal pole, however, the union rate decreases to around 60 % [2, 4, 10]. In a single-center study comparing outcomes with and without AVN, Chang et al. [2] reported that union occurred in 71 % of patients with proximal pole scaphoid nonunion, but only 50 % of patients with nonunion and AVN. Risk factors associated with failure of this vascularized bone graft included preoperative humpback deformity, female gender, older age, avascularity of the proximal pole, nonscrew fixation of the graft, and the use of tobacco.

In the presence of AVN and a humpback deformity (defined as a lateral intrascaphoid angle more than 45 °), a larger structural graft, such as a free medial femoral condyle flap, may be more appropriate to ensure fracture union [11, 12]. Unlike the 1,2 ICSRA vascularized bone graft, which is limited in size, the medial femoral condyle flap has sufficient structural support to correct the humpback deformity and restore carpal geometry. Jones et al. compared the outcomes of 1,2 ICSRA and medial femoral condyle in the management of scaphoid nonunion with carpal collapse and avascularity of the proximal pole [11]. The authors noted that patients treated with the 1,2 ICSRA graft had a 60 % union rate compared to a 100 % union rate (13 of 13 patients) within the medial femoral condyle cohort.

References

1. Kakar S, Bishop AT, Shin AY. Role of vascularized bone grafts in the treatment of scaphoid nonunions associated with proximal pole avascular necrosis and carpal collapse. J Hand Surg. 2011;36:722–5.
2. Chang MA, Bishop AT, Moran SL, Shin AY. The outcomes and complications of 1,2 intercompartmental supraretinacular artery pedicled vascularized bone grafting of scaphoid nonunions. J Hand Surg. 2006;31A:387–96.
3. Schmitt R Christopoulos G, Wagner H, et al. Avascular necrosis (AVN) of the proximal fragment in scaphoid nonunion: is intravenous contrast agent necessary in MRI? Eur J Radiol. 2011;77:222–7.
4. Straw RG, Davis TRC, Dias JJ. Scaphoid nonunion: treatment with a pedicled vascularized bone graft based on the 1,2-intercompartmental supraretinacular branch of the radial artery. J Hand Surg. 2002;27B:413–6.
5. Amadio PC, Taleisnik J. Fractures of the carpal bones. In: Green DP, editor. Operative hand surgery. Vol 1. Philadelphia: Elsevier Churchill Livingstone, 1999. pp. 809–69.
6. Zaidemberg C, Siebert JW, Angrigiani C. A new vascularized bone graft for scaphoid nonunion. J Hand Surg. 1991;16A:474–8.

7. Uerpairojkit C, Leechavengvongs S, Witoonchart K. Primary vascularized distal radius bone graft for nonunion of the scaphoid. J Hand Surg. 2000;25B:266–270.

8. Malizos KN, Dailiana ZH, Kirou M, Vragalas V, Xenakis TA, Soucacos PN. Longstanding nonunions of scaphoid fractures with bone loss: successful reconstruction with vascularized bone grafts. J Hand Surg. 2001;26B:330–4.

9. Tsai TT, Chao EK, Tu YK, Chen AC, Lee MS, Ueng SW. Management of scaphoid nonunion with avascular necrosis using 1,2-intercompartmental supraretinacular arterial bone grafts. Chang Gung Med J. 2002;25:321–328.

10. Boyer MI, von Schroeder HP, Axelrod TS. Scaphoid nonunion with avascular necrosis of the proximal pole: treatment with a vascularized bone graft from the dorsum of the distal radius. J Hand Surg. 1998;23B:686–90.

11. Jones DB Jr, Burger H, Bishop AT, Shin AY. Treatment of scaphoid waist nonunions with an avascular proximal pole and carpal collapse. A comparison of two vascularized bone grafts. J Bone Joint Surg Am. 2008;90:2616–25.

12. Higgins JP, Burger HK. Proximal scaphoid arthroplasty using the medial femoral trochlea flap. J Wrist Surg. 2013;2:228–33.

Chapter 14
Dorsal Capsular-Based Vascularized Distal Radius Graft for Scaphoid Nonunion

Loukia K. Papatheodorou and Dean G. Sotereanos

Case Presentation

A 27-year-old right-hand dominant manual laborer was referred to our clinic with a 7-month history of persistent right radial wrist pain after a fall onto his outstretched hand. He was initially diagnosed with a proximal pole scaphoid fracture and treated with a removable short-arm thumb spica splint. The patient denied tobacco use, and his prior medical history was noncontributory.

Physical Assessment

At the time of presentation, the patient had mild swelling over the dorsum of the right wrist and marked tenderness to direct palpation in the anatomic snuffbox. Wrist extension was 70° with pain, and wrist flexion was 60° with pain. Sensation was intact in the median, radial, and ulnar nerve distributions. Motor strength was 5/5 in all

D. G. Sotereanos (✉) · L. K. Papatheodorou
Department of Orthopaedic Surgery, University of Pittsburgh,
Pittsburgh, PA, USA
e-mail: dsoterea@hotmail.com

University of Pittsburgh Medical Center, Pittsburgh, PA, USA

© Springer International Publishing Switzerland 2015   157
J. Yao (ed.), *Scaphoid Fractures and Nonunions*,
DOI 10.1007/978-3-319-18977-2_14

Fig. 14.1 Anteroposterior (*AP*) radiograph of the *right* wrist showing a nonunion of the proximal pole of the scaphoid. (Published with kind permission from ©Loukia K. Papatheodorou and Dean G. Sotereanos, 2015. All Rights Reserved)

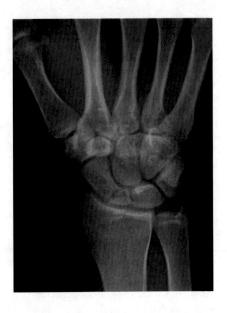

distributions except wrist extension and wrist flexion, which were graded 4/5 secondary to pain.

Diagnostic Studies/Diagnosis

Radiographs of the right wrist including scaphoid views revealed a scaphoid nonunion of the proximal pole with sclerosis (Fig. 14.1). Magnetic resonance imaging of the right wrist confirmed the diagnosis of avascular necrosis of the proximal pole of the scaphoid (Fig. 14.2).

Management Options

Scaphoid proximal pole fractures are more prone to nonunion than the more distal fractures because of the tenuous vascularity of the proximal part of the scaphoid, due to the retrograde interosseous

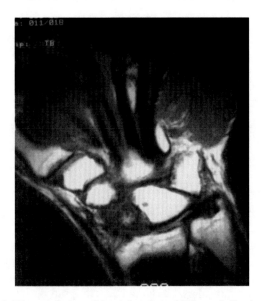

Fig. 14.2 T1 coronal view of the *right* wrist on MRI scan indicating avascular necrosis of the proximal fragment of the scaphoid. (Published with kind permission from ©Loukia K. Papatheodorou and Dean G. Sotereanos, 2015. All Rights Reserved)

blood supply of the scaphoid [1]. Moreover, the proximal pole of the scaphoid is most susceptible to avascular necrosis, which further impairs healing [2]. Treatment of proximal pole scaphoid nonunions with evidence of avascular necrosis is a challenging problem. The main complication of treatment is persistent non-union. Preoperative risk factors for nonunion include smoking, history of previous surgical procedures, the presence of humpback deformity, or carpal collapse. If a scaphoid nonunion is left untreat-ed, the wrist often undergoes progressive degenerative changes culminating in scaphoid nonunion advanced collapse.

Several treatment options have been proposed for the man-agement of scaphoid proximal pole nonunions accompanied by avascular necrosis, including excision of the scaphoid proximal pole, open reduction and internal fixation with or without nonvas-cularized bone graft, and vascularized bone graft. Although the reported union rate with the use of nonvascularized bone grafts ranges from 80 to 94%, the rate drops to 47% in the presence of avascular necrosis of the proximal pole [3, 4]. Vascularized bone grafts have demonstrated superior biologic and mechanical properties, improving the viability of the scaphoid proximal pole and leading to a more favorable outcome and a higher union rate (88–91%) than conventional bone grafts [3, 4]. The choice of vascularized bone graft depends on the location and the deformity of the scaphoid nonunion.

Management Chosen

For this patient with a scaphoid proximal pole nonunion accompanied by avascular necrosis but without humpback deformity and without carpal collapse, we utilized a capsular-based vascularized bone graft from the dorsal distal radius. This graft is nourished by the fourth extensor compartment artery, allowing easy access to the scaphoid proximal pole with a short arc of rotation minimizing the risk of nutrient vessel kinking [5, 6].

Surgical Technique

The procedure is performed under general anesthesia, tourniquet control, and loupe magnification. Regional anesthesia can also be applied. A 4-cm straight dorsal incision centered just ulnar to the Lister's tubercle is performed. Dissection is carried through the subcutaneous tissues. The extensor retinaculum of the fourth dorsal compartment is partially released to expose the wrist capsule and the distal radius. The extensor pollicis longus tendon is identified and retracted radially, and the extensor digitorum communis tendons are retracted ulnarly.

Next, the capsular-based vascularized distal radius graft is outlined with a skin marker on the dorsal wrist capsule. The flap is trapezoidal in shape with the length approximately 2 cm and is widened from 1 cm at the radial bone block to 1.5 cm at its metacarpal

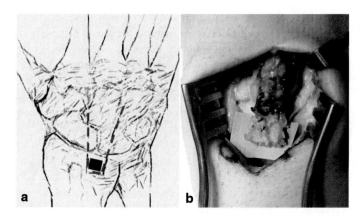

Fig. 14.3 Schematic **a** and operative view **b** of the dorsal capsular-based vascularized distal radius graft. The capsular graft is outlined with *red dotted* line, and the bone graft is marked with *black* color. (Published with kind permission from ©Loukia K. Papatheodorou and Dean G. Sotereanos, 2015. All Rights Reserved)

base (Fig. 14.3). The capsular flap is outlined sharply with a knife. The bone graft is harvested from the distal aspect of the dorsal radius just ulnar and distal to Lister's tubercle sized approximately 1 × 1 cm including the dorsal ridge of the distal radius (Fig. 14.3). The bone graft is outlined on the distal radius cortex with multiple drill holes by using a 1.0-mm side-cutting drill bit. The graft is elevated with a thin osteotome, with care taken to maintain 2–3 mm of the distal radius cortex intact to minimize the risk of propagation onto the articular cartilage of the radiocarpal joint. The depth of the bone block is approximately 7 mm. The capsular flap is elevated along with the bone graft from the underlying tissues in a proximal-to-distal direction with care to prevent detachment of the dorsal scapholunate ligament.

Once the flap was elevated, attention is directed toward the scaphoid. The scaphoid proximal pole nonunion site is identified by flexing the wrist. The cartilage shell in this patient was not grossly disrupted, and the nonunion site was not violated. Fixation of the nonunion was performed under fluoroscopic control. Two 1-mm smooth Kirschner wires were inserted from the proximal pole of the scaphoid oriented toward the base of the thumb with the wrist in extreme flexion. One of these served as a guide wire for a cannulated screw and the other served as a derotational wire. Care was taken to place the guide wire for the screw perpendicular to the fracture site and as volar as possible, while maintaining sufficient purchase of the proximal and distal fragments. The headless compression screw was inserted and buried underneath the articular surface by approximately 2 mm, and the derotational wire was then removed.

Once the fracture nonunion was secured, a dorsal trough was created across the nonunion site with a side-cutting burr in a nonarticular location. All nonvascular nonviable tissue was curetted out and excavated from the nonunion site. A microsuture anchor was placed at the floor of the trough to avoid dislodgement of the graft. Then, the graft with its capsular attachment was gently inserted into the scaphoid trough with minimal rotation (10–30°) due to the close proximity of the graft donor site. The graft was secured with a mattress stitch, from the suture anchor, through the perimeter of the graft periosteum. Care was taken to tie this stitch over the graft without compressing the pedicle. Hemostasis was obtained, the wound was irrigated, and the incision was closed with 3–0 nylon sutures.

Clinical Course and Outcome

Postoperatively, a short-arm thumb spica splint with the wrist in neutral position was applied for 2 weeks, followed by a short-arm thumb spica cast for another 4 weeks. Then, a removable forearm-based thumb spica splint was used until solid union occurred. Radiographs were obtained with the cast removed in 6 weeks and monthly thereafter to assess union progression. Solid bone union was achieved at 10 weeks after surgery. The immobilization period was followed by physiotherapy to restore the range of motion of the wrist and the grip strength. The patient returned to his previous activities as manual laborer at 5 months postoperatively.

At his 24-month follow-up visit, the patient was free of right wrist pain. He had full pronation and supination and a minor lack

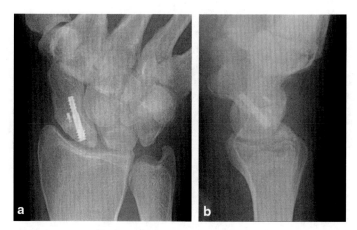

Fig. 14.4 AP **a** and lateral **b** radiographs of the *right* wrist joint at 24 months postoperatively showing no evidence of scaphoid necrosis or arthritic changes of the radiocarpal joint. Note the bone anchor next to the cannulated screw. (Published with kind permission from ©Loukia K. Papatheodorou and Dean G. Sotereanos, 2015. All Rights Reserved)

of wrist flexion and extension of 10°. The grip strength was normal, and the Mayo Modified Wrist Score was excellent (100/100). Radiographic evaluation of right wrist revealed no signs of scaphoid necrosis or arthritic changes of the radiocarpal joint (Fig. 14.4). No arthritic changes were noted at the dorsal ridge of the radius, where the graft had been harvested.

Clinical Pearls/Pitfalls

- Leave intact 2–3 mm of the distal radius cortex to minimize the risk of an intra-articular fracture.
- Elevate the capsular flap gently with care to prevent detachment of the dorsal scapholunate ligament.
- Full wrist flexion facilitates scaphoid proximal pole exposure.
- Destabilizing the nonunion can make the fixation more challenging.

- Insert 2 Kirschner wires from the proximal pole toward the base of the thumb. One serves as a derotational wire.
- Place a screw that is 6 mm shorter than measured, to prevent penetration of the distal articular surface.
- In cases with a very small fragment of the proximal pole, consider a mini Herbert cannulated screw.
- Place the graft in the excavated cavity of the proximal pole in cases with a very small fragment.
- Secure the graft with a microsuture anchor to avoid dislodgment in the early postoperative period.
- This technique is contraindicated for scaphoid nonunion with humpback deformity or scaphoid nonunion advanced collapse wrist stage II or greater.

Literature Review and Discussion

We have utilized the capsular-based vascularized distal radius graft for scaphoid nonunions since 2000. Our clinical series includes 53 patients with proximal pole scaphoid nonunion 41 with avascular necrosis [5, 6]. The mean patient age was 28 years (range, 19–43 years) and an average time from injury to surgery of 22 months. At a mean time of 13.6 weeks (range, 6–24 weeks) postoperatively, solid union was achieved in 46 of 53 patients (87%). Thirty-six out of 41 patients with avascular necrosis of the proximal pole healed their nonunions. Six patients had persistent nonunion and one fibrous union as determined by computed tomography scan. Forty of the patients with solid bone union were completely pain free and six complained of slight pain with strenuous activities. Wrist range of motion and grip strength were improved significantly after surgery. With a minimum follow-up of 1 year, no arthritic changes were noted at the dorsal ridge of the radius. No donor site morbidity was observed.

Our results compare favorably with others reported in the literature. A meta-analysis demonstrated an overall union rate of 88% with vascularized bone grafts for scaphoid nonunion with an avascular proximal pole [3]. In this study, a variety of techniques were used including free vascularized iliac crest grafts, vascular bundle implantation, and vascularized bone graft based on the first dorsal metacarpal artery. In another meta-analysis, the reported union rate was 91 % with the use of vascularized bone grafts in patients with prior failed surgery and/or avascular necrosis of proximal pole [4].

There are several published series with good-to-excellent results with the use of the vascularized bone graft from distal radius based on the 1,2 intercompartmental supraretinacular artery (1,2 ICSRA) [7–11]. In a large series with 48 patients with scaphoid nonunion, solid union was achieved in 34 patients [10]. Of the 24 nonunions with an avascular proximal pole, only 12 went to union (50 %). The authors used various techniques of fixation (Kirschner wires, cannulated screws, no fixation of the graft) and they found that screw fixation had better union rate than the other techniques.

In another study with 30 patients with scaphoid nonunion, 11 proximal poles with avascular necrosis, the reported union rate was 93 % using the 1,2 ICSRA graft [11]. The authors used cannulated screw fixation and performed a concomitant radial styloidectomy in all patients to decrease tension on the vascular pedicle. We believe that this measure was the key element for their reported high union rate since the 1,2 ICSRA graft needs to be rotated almost 180° to reach the nonunion site. A surgeon should consider performing a radial styloidectomy to avoid tension on the vascular pedicle, a step that is not necessary with the capsular-based graft.

In summary, the dorsal capsular-based vascularized distal radius graft for proximal pole scaphoid nonunion is a simple technique and permits expedient harvesting without the need for dissection of small-caliber vessels or microsurgical anastomoses. It is harvested from a position that allows easy access to the proximal scaphoid pole, and the short arc of rotation lessens the risk of vascular impairment caused by kinking of the nutrient vessel. Based on our experience, this graft provides successful clinical outcomes with regard to both union rate and postoperative wrist range of motion with minimal donor site morbidity.

References

1. Gelberman RH, Menon J. The vascularity of the scaphoid bone. J Hand Surg Am 1980;5:508–13
2. Simonian PT, Trumble TE. Scaphoid Nonunion. J Am Acad Orthop Surg 1994;2:185–91
3. Merrell GA, Wolfe SW, Slade JF 3rd. Treatment of scaphoid nonunions: quantitative meta-analysis of the literature. J Hand Surg Am 2002;27:685–91
4. Munk B, Larsen CF. Bone grafting the scaphoid nonunion: a systematic review of 147 publications including 5,246 cases of scaphoid nonunion. Acta Orthop Scand 2004;75:618–29
5. Sotereanos DG, Darlis NA, Dailiana ZH, Sarris IK, Malizos KN. A capsular-based vascularized distal radius graft for proximal pole scaphoid pseudarthrosis. J Hand Surg Am 2006;31:580–7
6. Venouziou AI, Sotereanos DG. Supplemental graft fixation for distal radius vascularized bone graft. J Hand Surg Am 2012;37:1475–79
7. Zaidemberg C, Siebert JW, Angrigiani C. A new vascularized bone graft for scaphoid nonunion. J Hand Surg Am 1991;16:474–8
8. Boyer MI, von Schroeder HP, Axelrod TS. Scaphoid nonunion with avascular necrosis of the proximal pole. Treatment with a vascularized bone graft from the dorsum of the distal radius. J Hand Surg Br 1998;23:686–90
9. Malizos KN, Zachos V, Dailiana ZH, Zalavras C, Varitimidis S, Hantes M, Karantanas A. Scaphoid nonunions: management with vascularized bone grafts from the distal radius: a clinical and functional outcome study. Plast Reconstr Surg 2007;119:1513–25
10. Chang MA, Bishop AT, Moran SL, Shin AY. The outcomes and complications of 1,2-intercompartmental supraretinacular artery pedicled vascularized bone grafting of scaphoid nonunions. J Hand Surg Am 2006;31:387–96
11. Waitayawinyu T, McCallister WV, Katolik LI, Schlenker JD, Trumble TE. Outcome after vascularized bone grafting of scaphoid nonunions with avascular necrosis. J Hand Surg Am 2009;34:387–94

Chapter 15
Scaphoid Nonunion: Surgical Fixation with Vascularized Bone Grafts–Volar Pedicle

Christophe Mathoulin, Mathilde Gras

Case Presentation

A 42-year-old man presented with wrist pain that had been on going for several months. His history revealed that he had fallen 14 months previously. At that point, X-rays showed a scaphoid fracture, which was treated with a simple cast for 2 months. The patient subsequently had disabling pain. New X-rays showed a scaphoid nonunion with bone resorption and humpback scaphoid deformity.

Physical Assessment/Diagnosis

- The pain score was 8 on the VAS scale.
- Extension was 50° versus 80°on the opposite side.
- Flexion was 55° versus 80° on the opposite side.
- Radial deviation was 15° versus 25° on the opposite side.
- Ulnar deviation was 20° versus 40° on the opposite side.

C. Mathoulin(✉)
Institut de la Main, Hand department, Clinique Jouvenet, 6 Square Jouvenet, Paris 75016, France
e-mail: cmathoulin@orange.fr

M. Gras
Department of Hand Surgery, Institute de la Main, Clinique Jouvenet, association loi 1901 sise 6 square Jouvenet, Paris 75016, France

© Springer International Publishing Switzerland 2015
J. Yao (ed.), *Scaphoid Fractures and Nonunions*,
DOI 10.1007/978-3-319-18977-2_15

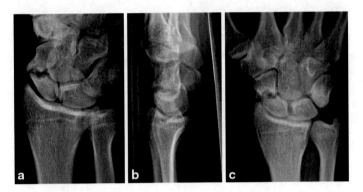

Fig. 15.1 a, b, c X-rays of scaphoid nonunion, with central bone loss and adaptative DISI. (Published with kind permission of © Christophe Mathoulin and Mathilde Gras, 2015. All Rights Reserved)

- Full pronation and supination
- Grip strength was 25 kgf versus 55 kgf on the opposite side.
- DASH score was 56.82.
- X-rays (Fig. 15.1a, b, c) showed nonunion at the scaphoid waist with bone resorption (type D3 in Herbert's classification) along with an adaptive DISI. There were no signs of necrosis.

Management Chosen

It was decided to treat this patient with a vascularized bone graft utilizing a volar pedicled graft based off the volar carpal artery. The patient was informed that smoking was not allowed before and after surgery.

Surgical Procedure

The surgery was performed under regional anesthesia as an outpatient procedure through a single volar incision.

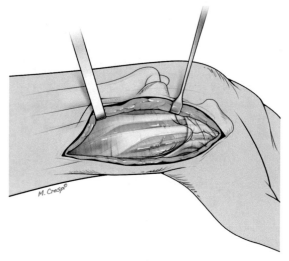

Fig. 15.2 Drawing showing the volar lateral approach for scaphoid. (Published with kind permission of © Christophe Mathoulin and Mathilde Gras, 2015. All Rights Reserved)

First Step: Exploration and Preparation of the Nonunion

The classic volar Henry approach was extended distally toward the distal scaphoid tubercle and the capsule was opened (Fig. 15.2). The two ends of scaphoid were cleaned and any fibrosis excised. The scaphoid showed a humpback deformity. Reduction was performed with an osteotome and fixed with temporary K-wires.

Second Step: Graft Harvesting

The graft was harvested from the distal and ulnar aspects of the volar radius. The volar carpal artery is always located in the volar periosteum of the radius, just distal to the distal part of the superficial aponeurosis of the pronator quadratus. The superficial aponeurosis was opened over its last distal centimeter; the muscle was retracted and then temporarily fixed with a K-wire. The periosteum was sectioned longitudinally on the distal edge of the radius where the superficial aponeurosis of the pronator quadratus

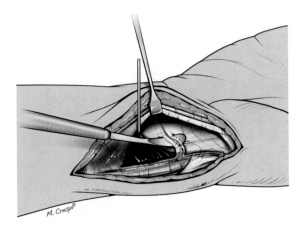

Fig. 15.3 Drawing showing the pedicle elevated with the periosteum on the radial side. (Published with kind permission of © Christophe Mathoulin and Mathilde Gras, 2015. All Rights Reserved)

ends on the radius. The pedicle was elevated with the periosteum on the radial side (Fig. 15.3). The structural bone graft was harvested from the radius with an osteotome and shaped as a pyramid to fit perfectly in the scaphoid defect and to avoid any detachment of the periosteum and pedicle from the graft (Fig. 15.4). The pedicle was dissected up to the radial artery, where the volar carpal artery originates (Fig. 15.5).

Third Step: Fixation

The scaphoid was fixed with a retrograde cannulated headless compression screw (Fig. 15.6). In this case, however, the graft was not sufficiently compressed between both ends of the scaphoid. To rectify this, a K-wire was inserted parallel to the screw, a bit more volar, to capture and to fix the graft to the scaphoid (Fig. 15.7). The capsule was sutured without compressing the pedicle.

A palmar splint was worn by the patient until bone union was achieved 45 days later. Physical therapy started immediately after union.

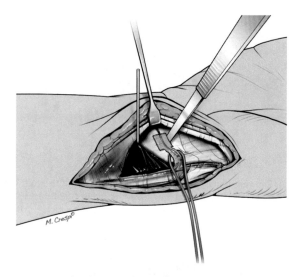

Fig. 15.4 Drawing showing the harvesting of bone graft from the radius with an osteotome. (Published with kind permission of © Christophe Mathoulin and Mathilde Gras, 2015. All Rights Reserved)

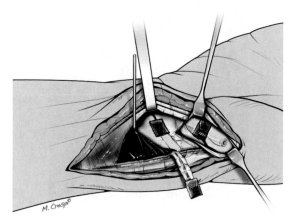

Fig. 15.5 Drawing showing the pedicle dissected up to the radial artery, where the volar carpal artery originates. (Published with kind permission of © Christophe Mathoulin and Mathilde Gras, 2015. All Rights Reserved)

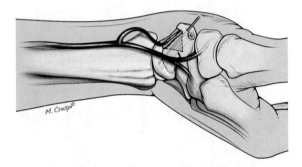

Fig. 15.6 Drawing showing the principles of placement of the graft into the volar bone loss of scaphoid nonunion, fixed by screw. (Published with kind permission of © Christophe Mathoulin and Mathilde Gras, 2015. All Rights Reserved)

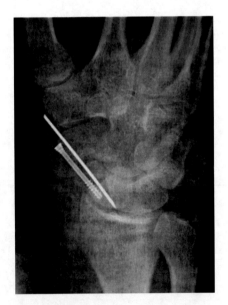

Fig. 15.7 Postoperative X-rays. (Published with kind permission of © Christophe Mathoulin and Mathilde Gras, 2015. All Rights Reserved)

Clinical Course and Outcome

- Bone union was achieved at 6 weeks (Fig. 15.8).
- At 2 years, the adaptive DISI had totally disappeared and the scaphoid was solid (Fig. 15.9a,b).
- The pain score was 0 on the VAS scale.
- Extension was 70° versus 80°on the opposite side
- Flexion was 65° versus 80° on the opposite side
- Radial deviation was 25° versus 25° on the opposite side
- Ulnar deviation was 40° versus 40° on the opposite side
- Full pronation and supination
- Grip strength was 50 kgf versus 55 kgf on the opposite side.

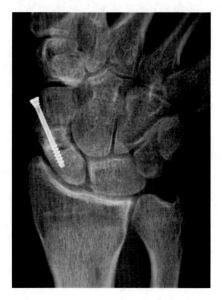

Fig. 15.8 X-rays at 45 days after K-wire removal. (Published with kind permission of © Christophe Mathoulin and Mathilde Gras, 2015. All Rights Reserved)

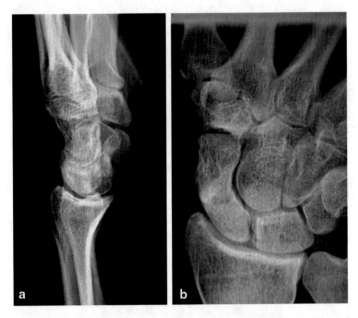

Fig. 15.9 a, b X-rays after 2 years showing a complete reconstruction of scaphoid with corrected DISI. (Published with kind permission of © Christophe Mathoulin and Mathilde Gras, 2015. All Rights Reserved)

Clinical Pearls/Pitfalls

- Fixation is done with a retrograde cannulated screw.
- The pedicle has to be dissected up to the radial artery to provide good graft mobilization; it is important not to damage this pedicle.
- The proximal, medial, and distal sides of the graft are harvested with a 1 cm osteotome; a smaller one (0.5 cm) is used for the lateral side. The pedicle is gently elevated when the bone cuts are performed.
- The graft should be pyramid-shaped to prevent the periosteum from separating from the graft and to maintain good graft vascularity. The shape of scaphoid defect is almost always pyramidal, particularly after reduction of a humpback deformity.
- The distal side of the graft is harvested with the osteotome in an oblique bone cut to avoid intra-articular fracture of the radius.

- The patient has to agree to stop smoking before and after surgery until to obtain union.

Literature Review and Discussion

The scaphoid is poorly vascularized and the treatment of scaphoid nonunion remains controversial. Classical nonvascularized bone grafts are still the gold standard, but nonunion persists in 6–23 % of cases according to Merrell's meta-analysis [1]. Union was achieved in 47 % of cases in the proximal pole with wedge grafting and screw fixation and in 88 % of cases when a vascularized bone graft was used. Munk and Larsen [2] also found a better union rate with vascularized bone grafts (91 %, range 87–94) than nonvascularized bone grafts with fixation (84 %, range 82–85).

In our own study with vascularized bone grafts [3], union was achieved in 96 % of cases of primary treatment and 89.5 % in patients undergoing secondary treatment. Our technique of harvesting a vascularized bone graft pedicled on the volar carpal artery from the volar distal radius is performed through a single incision. The volar carpal artery was present in all cadaveric dissections that we have performed (Fig. 15.10) [4].

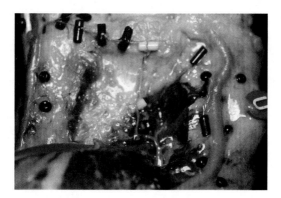

Fig. 15.10 Cadaveric dissection showing the vascular "T" with the volar carpal artery (red), the branch from ulnar artery (blue), and the final volar interosseous artery (yellow). (Published with kind permission of © Christophe Mathoulin and Mathilde Gras, 2015. All Rights Reserved)

Vascularized bone grafts seem to be a good option for primary treatment of scaphoid nonunion because the union rate is very high. This case illustrates the use of a vascularized bone graft based off the volar carpal artery. This technique can be carried out in an outpatient setting using regional anesthesia and a single volar incision.

References

1. Merrell GA, Wolfe SW, Slade JF. Treatment of scaphoid non-unions: quantitative meta-analysis of the literature. J Hand Surg Am. 2002;27(4):685–91.
2. Munk B, Larsen CF. Bone grafting the scaphoid nonunion: a systematic review of 147 publications including 5246 cases of scaphoid nonunion. Acta Orthop Scand. 2004;75(5): 618–29.
3. Gras M, Mathoulin M. Vascularized bone graft pedicled on the volar carpal artery from the volar distal radius as primary procedure for scaphoid non-union. Orthop Traumatol: Surg Res. 2011;97:800–6
4. Mathoulin C, Haerle M. Vascularized bone graft from the palmar carpal artery for treatment of scaphoid non-union. J Hand Surg [Am] 1998;23B:318–23.

Chapter 16
Scaphoid Nonunion: Surgical Fixation with Vascularized Bone Graft–Free Medial Femoral Condyle Graft

Peter C. Rhee and Alexander Y. Shin

Case Presentation

The patient is an 18-year-old, right-hand-dominant, active duty soldier with a chief complaint of left radial-sided wrist pain after falling from his bunk onto an outstretched left hand approximately 5 months prior. He initially attributed the pain to a wrist "sprain" and did not seek medical attention. He has had progressive increase in radial-sided wrist pain with inability to perform push-ups and marked limitation in wrist motion that inhibited him from performing his work duties. The use of a removal thumb spica brace has given him minimal relief.

P. C. Rhee (✉)
F. Edward Hebert School of Medicine, USUHS, Bethesda, MD, USA
e-mail: peter.c.rhee@me.com

Department of Orthopedic Surgery and Rehabilitation, San Antonio Military Medical Center, Fort Sam Houston, San Antonio, TX, USA

A. Y. Shin
Department of Orthopedic Surgery, Mayo Clinic, Rochester, MN, USA

© Springer International Publishing Switzerland 2015
J. Yao (ed.), *Scaphoid Fractures and Nonunions,*
DOI 10.1007/978-3-319-18977-2_16

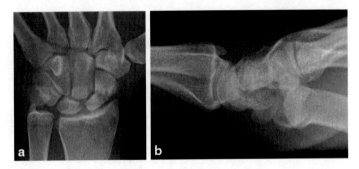

Fig. 16.1 Plain radiographs of the *left* wrist. Posteroanterior **a** and lateral **b**. (Published with kind permission of © Peter C. Rhee and Alexander Y. Shin, 2015. All Rights Reserved)

Physical Assessment

On examination, the patient's left wrist had radial-sided soft tissue edema with tenderness to palpation at the distal scaphoid tubercle, pain with axial loading of the 1st ray, and discomfort to deep pressure at the anatomic snuffbox. Wrist range of motion was as follows (left/right): flexion 30°/65°, extension 20°/70°, radial deviation 5°/15°, and ulnar deviation 20°/30°. Grip strength was reduced in the left (20 kg) compared to the right (50 kg). There was a positive scaphoid shift test which elicited pain, but not instability.

Diagnostic Studies

Wrist radiographs were obtained that revealed a scaphoid waist nonunion and dorsal intercalated segmental instability (DISI) pattern of the lunate (radiolunate angle 31°) without radioscaphoid or midcarpal arthrosis (Fig. 16.1a, b). A computed tomography (CT) scan confirmed bone resorption at the nonunion site, proximal pole sclerosis [1], and scaphoid foreshortening or the so-called humpback deformity (lateral intra-scaphoid angle of 70°, Fig. 16.2a, b) [2].

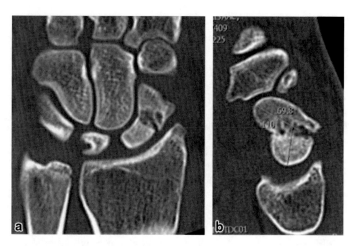

Fig. 16.2 Computed tomography of the *left* wrist. Coronal **a** and sagittal **b** reformats. (Published with kind permission of © Peter C. Rhee and Alexander Y. Shin, 2015. All Rights Reserved)

Diagnosis

Left scaphoid waist nonunion with scaphoid foreshortening, carpal collapse, and probable avascular necrosis (AVN) of the proximal pole.

Management Options

Due to the patient's young age, absence of degenerative change within the wrist, and carpal collapse, he was recommended a scaphoid waist nonunion debridement, bone grafting, and rigid fixation. In the absence of proximal pole AVN, bone grafting options included cancellous bone (distal radius or iliac crest) [3], bone substitute (beta-tricalcium phosphate and calcium sulfate) [4], and corticocancellous bone (distal radius or iliac crest) [5]. In the presence of proximal pole AVN, bone grafting options included nonvascularized interposition bone graft with arteriovenous (AV) bundle implantation [6], pedicled vascularized corticocancellous bone graft (thumb metacarpal, or dorsal and volar distal radius) [7–9], or free vascularized corticocancellous bone graft (iliac crest or medial femoral condyle) [10, 11].

Management Chosen

The patient agreed with the recommended surgical plan and the necessity of a structural bone graft, due to the scaphoid "humpback" deformity and bone resorption. The utilization of a nonvascularized iliac crest corticocancellous bone graft versus a vascularized free medial femoral condyle (MFC) corticocancellous bone graft would be dictated upon the intra-operative findings of proximal pole vascularity, defined by the presence or absence (AVN) of punctate bleeding from the proximal pole of the scaphoid after nonunion debridement and release of the tourniquet [12]. However, if the proximal pole of the scaphoid was noted to be fragmented or devoid of cartilage intra-operatively, a salvage procedure in the form of a scaphoid excision and four corner arthrodesis would be performed.

After the induction of general anesthesia, the patient was positioned supine with the affected arm draped free on a hand table. The entire ipsilateral lower extremity was prepped and draped up toward the flank to allow for iliac crest or MFC bone graft harvest. A well-padded bump was placed distally under the drapes to maintain knee flexion and external rotation of the hip which can greatly improve visualization and exposure during harvest of the free MFC graft [13].

After the exsanguination of the left upper extremity and tourniquet inflation, an extended volar Russe-type approach to the scaphoid was performed. The scaphoid nonunion site was exposed, and the fibrous interposed tissue was debrided. A microsagittal saw was used to create flat bone surfaces with minimal resection of bone. The proximal pole was sclerotic and appeared similar to ivory on inspection, and release of the tourniquet confirmed no bleeding from the proximal pole or the scaphoid waist fragment at the nonunion surface (Fig. 16.3a). However, no cartilage loss was noted at

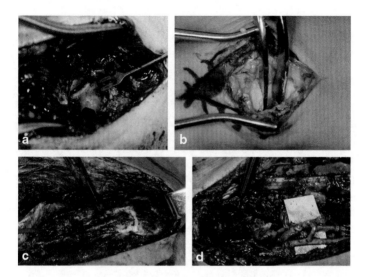

Fig. 16.3 Intraoperative images. Lack of punctate bleeding from the proximal pole of the scaphoid **a**, scaphoid over distraction with the lamina spreader **b**, free medial femoral condyle harvest **c**, and insetting of the vascularized bone graft **d**. (Published with kind permission of © Peter C. Rhee and Alexander Y. Shin, 2015. All Rights Reserved)

the proximal pole of the scaphoid, the radial styloid, or the scaphoid fossa.

The dense intramedullary bone was excavated from both fragments with curettes to remove the sclerotic bone and to produce a cavitary space into which cancellous bone graft could be packed later on. The DISI deformity was corrected with wrist hyperflexion and confirmed on fluoroscopy by a lunate in neutral position and was temporarily stabilized in this position with a percutaneous 0.0625 in. Kirschner wire driven from the dorsal distal radius into the lunate [13]. A lamina spreader was then placed into the nonunion site, and the proximal and distal scaphoid fragments were over-distracted to correct the scaphoid foreshortening and carpal collapse (Fig. 16.3b). A paper ruler was then used to measure the dimensions of the scaphoid waist bone void (width 10 mm, length 12 mm, and height 12 mm) to serve as a template for free MFC bone graft harvest.

The left lower extremity was gravity-exsanguinated and the sterile thigh tourniquet was inflated. A longitudinal incision (15 cm) was made extending from the medial tibial plateau proximally over the posterior border of the vastus medialis. The vastus medialis fascia was incised, and subfascial dissection was performed posteriorly while retracting the muscle belly anteriorly. The descending genicular artery (DGA) was identified proximally near the adductor hiatus and dissected distally toward the anastomoses of the osteoarticular branch of the DGA and the superior medial genicular artery (SMGA). The DGA was noted to be larger in diameter than the SMGA; therefore, it and the two accompanying vena comitantes were dissected off of the femur. The area of bone graft harvest was identified in the distal posterior aspect of the MFC, and the dimensions of the approximate bone graft size were marked over the harvest site. The pedicle was ligated, and the bone graft was harvested as described by Jones et al. (Fig. 16.3c) [14]. Additional cancellous bone graft was harvested after the removal of the free MFC bone graft and was packed into the cavitary defects within the two scaphoid fragments.

The free MFC graft was inset into the nonunion site (Fig. 16.3d), which was held open with the lamina spreader. The guide pin for the headless compression screw was inserted from the distal pole of the scaphoid in retrograde fashion. Fluoroscopy was used to confirm proper bone graft and guide pin positioning. After predrilling, the appropriately sized headless compression screw was implanted. There was no compression of the pedicle against the radial styloid; therefore, a radial styloidectomy was not performed. The DGA and one of its vena comitantes was anastomosed to the radial artery (end-to-side) and an accompanying vena comitantes (end-to-end) using microvascular technique. The incisions were closed with monofilament suture, and no attempt was made at repairing the radioscaphocapitate ligament.

Clinical Course and Outcome

The patient was placed into a postoperative long arm, thumb spica plaster splint with the wrist in neutral position. He was observed as an inpatient for pain control without vascular monitoring.

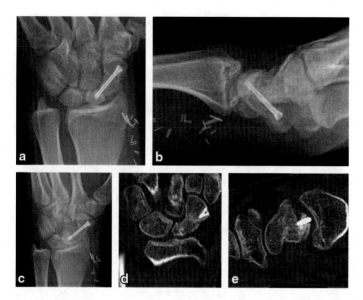

Fig. 16.4 Postoperative images. Posterioanterior **a**, lateral **b**, scaphoid view radiographs **c**. Coronal **d**, and sagittal **e** computed tomography reformats. (Published with kind permission of © Peter C. Rhee and Alexander Y. Shin, 2015. All Rights Reserved)

Microvascular anastomosis thromboprophylaxis consisted of enteric coated aspirin (325 mg) by mouth daily for 4 weeks. No weight bearing was allowed on the affected upper extremity. However, lower extremity weight bearing and knee range of motion was performed as tolerated immediately postoperative. A knee immobilizer and a single-arm crutch was utilized postoperative as needed and was weaned over a week period.

At 2 weeks postoperative, the sutures were removed and a thumb spica cast was applied for an additional 6 weeks. Plain radiographs at 6 weeks postoperative revealed consolidation of the free MFC graft into the native scaphoid with maintenance of neutral lunate position (Fig. 16.4a–c). A CT scan at 8 weeks postoperative confirmed bridging trabecular bone across the distal and proximal-free MFC bone graft junction sites (Fig. 16.4d, e). The patient was then placed into a removable, short arm, thumb spica brace for an additional 4 weeks until he was nontender to palpation at the anatomic snuffbox. At 4 months postoperative, the patient had no wrist or knee pain and affected wrist range of motion was flexion 50°, extension 60°, radial deviation 10°, and ulnar deviation 20°. He returned to performing push-ups and running 6 miles without discomfort.

Clinical Pearls/Pitfalls

- Scaphoid nonunions with "humpback" deformity, carpal collapse, and proximal pole AVN are indicated for free MFC VBG.
- Meticulous debridement of the nonunion site is integral to properly evaluate for AVN intra-operatively and for preparation for free MFC VBG.
- A lamina spreader can be utilized to over-distract the scaphoid to correct collapse and aids in insetting the free MFC VBG.
- In the setting of radial styloid beaking without complete radioscaphoid arthrosis (SNAC I), a radial styloidectomy can be performed in conjunction with the free MFC VBG.
- If the proximal pole of the scaphoid is small and at risk for fragmentation with insertion of a headless compression screw, utilize multiple K-wires for fixation.
- Lunate hyperextension (DISI) can be corrected with wrist flexion and temporary radiolunate transfixation with a K-wire prior to insetting of the free MFC VBG.
- Be prepared to perform a salvage procedure if radioscaphoid arthrosis is confirmed intra-operatively or if the proximal pole fractures with scaphoid fixation.

Literature Review and Discussion

The use of vascularized periosteum and bone from the MFC was initially described by Hertel and Masquelet as a pedicled flap based on the articular branch of the DGA or the SMGA for the treatment of lower extremity nonunions, segmental tibial bone loss, and revascularization in cases of aseptic necrosis about the knee [15]. In 1991, Doi et al. described the use of a free vascularized MFC corticoperiosteal onlay flap in addition to a vascularized MFC corticocancellous graft in the treatment of a variety of difficult nonunions [16]. The same author evolved the free MFC as a volar inlay graft for scaphoid nonunions [17] .

In the presence of proximal pole AVN, vascularized bone grafts (VBGs) are useful to revascularize the proximal pole and unite the scaphoid nonunion. It is postulated that the transplantation of viable osteocytes (greater than 90 % survival in transferred VBGs) can accelerate graft–host bone union through primary bone healing without resorption or creeping substitution [18–20]. Additionally, a canine model exhibited revascularization and active bone remodeling in proximal poles with AVN after VBG [21]. Both pedicled and free microvascular transferred bone grafts have been reported for use in scaphoid nonunions [6–11, 14].

The 1,2-intercompartmental supraretinacular artery (1,2-ICSRA)-pedicled distal radius graft is often employed for the treatment of scaphoid nonunions with AVN [22, 23]. The reported union rates range from 100 to 27 % in various studies [23–27]. Chang et al. reported an overall union rate of 71 % (34 of 48) in scaphoid nonunions that underwent VBG with the 1,2-ICSRA [5]. However, only 50 % (12 of 24) of scaphoids with proximal pole AVN united and 50 % (7 of 14) of failures occurred in patients with AVN and concomitant scaphoid foreshortening and/or DISI. Thus, the authors advised against the use of the 1,2-ICSRA VBG as a dorsal inlay graft when both AVN and scaphoid humpback deformity is present [8]. Similarly, Jones et al. reported a 40 % (4 of 10) union rate and inability to correct carpal collapse and alignment with use of the 1,2-ICSRA VBG [11].

The indication for free MFC VBG in the treatment of scaphoid nonunion is in the presence of associated scaphoid collapse, DISI deformity, and avascularity of the scaphoid which is confirmed intra-operatively as noted by the absence of punctate bleeding in a white sclerotic bone after release of the tourniquet [12]. Other relative indications include previously failed screw fixation or failed conventional nonvascularized wedge graft or the need for a large VBG (> 1.0 cm^3) [13]. The free MFC VBG can only be utilized if the proximal pole of the scaphoid has an intact cartilaginous shell, is of adequate size for fixation, and without fragmentation [11, 28]. If any of these characteristics are present, the patient should be considered for a salvage procedure (listed below) or a free medial femoral trochlea (MFT) osteocartilaginous VBG [29].

The contraindication for free MFC VBG is in the presence of radioscaphoid arthritis consistent with scaphoid nonunion advanced collapse (SNAC II or greater) in which case a salvage procedure such as a wrist denervation, scaphoid excision and four corner arthrodesis, proximal row carpectomy, or total wrist arthrodesis should be performed [13]. If radial styloid beaking (SNAC I) is present, a free MFC VBG can be performed with a supplementary radial styloidectomy. This procedure is not indicated for scaphoid nonunions with normal scaphoid geometry and AVN of the proximal pole or for ununited scaphoids with collapse but without evidence of AVN. In these cases, an inlay-pedicled VBG (1,2-ICSRA) or nonvascularized interposition structural bone graft may be performed, respectively [13].

The free MFC VBG can be utilized as a structural interposition graft combined with rigid headless compression screw fixation to restore scaphoid length and carpal alignment in nonunions complicated by both scaphoid foreshortening and proximal pole AVN [11, 28]. Doi et al. reported a 100% union rate at a mean of 12 weeks after surgery in ten patients with scaphoid nonunion secondary to AVN, suggested on magnetic resonance imaging (MRI) and confirmed intra-operatively, that underwent free MFC VBG without any long-term donor site morbidities [17]. Outcomes based on the Mayo Wrist Score were excellent in four patients, good in four patients, and fair in two patients with preoperative imaging studies exhibiting periscaphoid arthritis that had persistent postoperative pain [17]. Similarly, Jones et al. reported a 100% rate of union at a mean of 13 weeks after surgery in 12 patients with scaphoid nonunion with proximal pole AVN and carpal collapse [11]. There were significant improvements in scaphoid collapse (lateral intrascaphoid angle from 57° to 23°, $p < 0.001$) and carpal malalignment (scapholunate angle from 70 to 57° and radiolunate angle from 15 to 10°, $p = 0.05$ and $p = 0.03$, respectively). Postoperative mean wrist range of motion was flexion to 42° and extension to 40°

with a mean grip strength of 86 % (44 and 51 kg) compared to the unaffected hand. Although patients reported knee pain at the site of the MFC harvest for a mean of 6 weeks postoperative, there were no other donor site-related complications [11].

The optimal VBG is one that possesses structural integrity combined with a reliable and consistent pedicle that provides a robust blood supply and can be harvested with minimal donor site morbidity [11]. Scaphoid nonunions with proximal pole AVN and "humpback" deformity can be treated with a variety of techniques [3–11]. However, failure to address the structural and vascular deficiencies can result in poor outcomes [8, 11, 30]. The free MFC VBG provides an exuberant blood supply and stout corticocancellous bone that has displayed excellent union rates, correction of scaphoid geometry, restoration of carpal alignment, and promising clinical outcomes [11]. Therefore, it remains a valid surgical option in the treatment algorithm for scaphoid nonunions.

References

1. Smith ML, Bain GI, Chabrel N, Turner P, Carter C, Field J. Using computed tomography to assist with diagnosis of avascular necrosis complicating chronic scaphoid nonunion. J Hand Surg Am. 2009;34(6):1037–43.
2. Amadio PC, Berquist TH, Smith DK, Ilstrup DM, Cooney WP 3rd, Linscheid RL. Scaphoid malunion. J Hand Surg Am. 1989;14(4):679–87.
3. Cohen MS, Jupiter JB, Fallahi K, Shukla SK. Scaphoid waist nonunion with humpback deformity treated without structural bone graft. J Hand Surg Am. 2013;38(4):701–5.
4. Chu PJ, Shih JT. Arthroscopically assisted use of injectable bone graft substitutes for management of scaphoid nonunions. Arthroscopy. 2011;27(1):31–7.
5. Nakamura R, Horii E, Watanabe K, Tsunoda K, Miura T. Scaphoid nonunion: factors affecting the functional outcome of open reduction and wedge grafting with Herbert screw fixation. J Hand Surg. 1993;18(2):219–24.
6. Fernandez DL, Eggli S. Non-union of the scaphoid. Revascularization of the proximal pole with implantation of a vascular bundle and bone-grafting. J Bone Jt Surg. 1995;77A(6):883–93.
7. Bertelli JA, Tacca CP, Rost JR. Thumb metacarpal vascularized bone graft in long-standing scaphoid nonunion–a useful graft via dorsal or palmar approach: a cohort study of 24 patients. J Hand Surg Am. 2004;29(6):1089–97.

8. Chang MA, Bishop AT, Moran SL, Shin AY. The outcomes and complications of 1,2-intercompartmental supraretinacular artery pedicled vascularized bone grafting of scaphoid nonunions. J Hand Surg Am. 2006;31(3):387–96.

9. Gras M, Mathoulin C. Vascularized bone graft pedicled on the volar carpal artery from the volar distal radius as primary procedure for scaphoid nonunion. Orthop Traumatol Surg Res. 2011;97(8):800–6.

10. Arora R, Lutz M, Zimmermann R, Krappinger D, Niederwanger C, Gabl M. Free vascularised iliac bone graft for recalcitrant avascular nonunion of the scaphoid. J Bone Jt Surg Br. 2010;92(2):224–9.

11. Jones DB Jr, Burger H, Bishop AT, Shin AY. Treatment of scaphoid waist nonunions with an avascular proximal pole and carpal collapse. A comparison of two vascularized bone grafts. J Bone Jt Surg Am. 2008;90(12):2616–25.

12. Green DP. The effect of avascular necrosis on Russe bone grafting for scaphoid nonunion. J Hand Surg. 1985;10(5):597–605.

13. Rhee PC, Jones DB Jr, Bishop AT, Shin AY. Free medial femoral condyle vascularized bone grafting for scaphoid nonunions with proximal pole avascular necrosis and carpal collapse. Op Techn Orthop. 2012;22:159–66.

14. Jones DB Jr, Burger H, Bishop AT, Shin AY. Treatment of scaphoid waist nonunions with an avascular proximal pole and carpal collapse. Surgical technique. J Bone Jt Surg Am. 2009;91(Suppl 2):169–83.

15. Hertel R, Masquelet AC. The reverse flow medial knee osteoperiosteal flap for skeletal reconstruction of the leg. Description and anatomical basis. Surg Radiol Anat. 1989;11(4):257–62.

16. Sakai K, Doi K, Kawai S. Free vascularized thin corticoperiosteal graft. Plast Reconstr Surg. 1991;87(2):290–8.

17. Doi K, Oda T, Soo-Heong T, Nanda V. Free vascularized bone graft for nonunion of the scaphoid. J Hand Surg Am. 2000;25(3):507–19.

18. Dell PC, Burchardt H, Glowczewskie FP Jr. A roentgenographic, biomechanical, and histological evaluation of vascularized and non-vascularized segmental fibular canine autografts. J Bone Jt Surg. 1985;67(1):105–12 (American volume).

19. Shaffer JW, Field GA, Wilber RG, Goldberg VM. Experimental vascularized bone grafts: Histopathologic correlations with postoperative bone scan: the risk of flase positive results. J Orthop Res. 1987;5(3):311–9.

20. Goldberg VM, Shaffer JW, Field G, Davy DT. Biology of vascularized bone grafts. Orthop Clin N Am. 1987;18(2):197–205.

21. Sunagawa T, Bishop AT, Muramatsu K. Role of conventional and vascularized bone grafts in scaphoid nonunion with avascular necrosis: a canine experimental study [In Process Citation]. J Hand Surg. 2000;25(5):849–59 [MEDLINE record in process].

22. Sheetz KK, Bishop AT, Berger RA. The arterial blood supply of the distal radius and its potential use in vascularized pedicled bone grafts. J Hand Surg. 1995;20:902–14.

23. Steinmann SP, Bishop AT, Berger RA. Use of the 1,2 intercompartmental supraretinacular artery as a vascularized pedicle bone graft for difficult scaphoid nonunion. J Hand Surg Am. 2002;27(3):391–401.

24. Zaidemberg C, Siebert JW, Angrigiani C. A new vascularized bone graft for scaphoid nonunion. J Hand Surg Am. 1991;16(3):474–8.

25. Boyer MI, von Schroeder HP, Axelrod TS. Scaphoid nonunion with avascular necrosis of the proximal pole. Treatment with a vascularized bone graft from the dorsum of the distal radius. J Hand Surg Br. 1998;23(5):686–90.

26. Straw RG, Davis TR, Dias JJ. Scaphoid nonunion: treatment with a pedicled vascularized bone graft based on the 1,2 intercompartmental supraretinacular branch of the radial artery. J Hand Surg Br. 2002;27(5):413.

27. Uerpairojkit C, Leechavengvongs S, Witoonchart K. Primary vascularized distal radius bone graft for nonunion of the scaphoid. J Hand Surg Br. 2000;25(3):266–70.

28. Larson AN, Bishop AT, Shin AY. Free medial femoral condyle bone grafting for scaphoid nonunions with humpback deformity and proximal pole avascular necrosis. Tech Hand Up Extrem Surg. 2007;11(4):246–58.

29. Burger HK, Windhofer C, Gaggl AJ, Higgins JP. Vascularized medial femoral trochlea osteocartilaginous flap reconstruction of proximal pole scaphoid nonunions. J Hand Surg Am. 2013;38(4):690–700.

30. Merrell GA, Wolfe SW, Slade JF 3rd. Treatment of scaphoid nonunions: quantitative meta-analysis of the literature. J Hand Surg Am. 2002;27(4):685–91.

Chapter 17
Pediatric Scaphoid Nonunion

Joshua M. Abzug and Dan A. Zlotolow

Case Presentation

The patient is a 12-year-old right-hand-dominant male who in-jured his right wrist during a football game approximately 1 year prior to presentation. Initially, no medical treatment was sought; however, the patient had persistent limitation in motion as well as radial-sided wrist pain and therefore presented for further evalua-tion and treatment. The remainder of his past medical history was unremarkable.

Physical Assessment

The physical examination demonstrated tenderness to palpation about the right snuffbox. Additionally, the patient lacked 20° of wrist extension on the right side compared to the left. Wrist flex-ion and radial/ulnar deviation motions were symmetric. The re-mainder of the physical examination was unremarkable.

D. A. Zlotolow (✉)
Department of Orthopaedics, Temple University School of Medicine and Shriner's Hospital for Children Philadelphia, Philadelphia, PA, USA
e-mail: dzlotolow@yahoo.com

J. M. Abzug
Department of Orthopaedics, University of Maryland, Timonium, MD, USA

© Springer International Publishing Switzerland 2015　　　　191
J. Yao (ed.), *Scaphoid Fractures and Nonunions,*
DOI 10.1007/978-3-319-18977-2_17

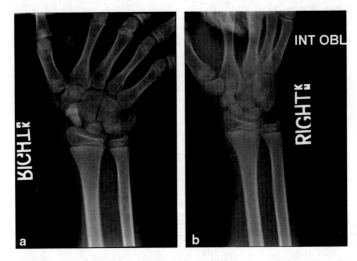

Fig. 17.1 a Posteroanterior and **b** internal oblique views of the *right* wrist demonstrating a scaphoid waist nonunion. (Courtesy of Shriner's Hospital for Children, Philadelphia, PA)

Diagnostic Studies

Plain radiographs demonstrated a nonunion of the scaphoid waist with the lunate in extension representing mild dorsal intercalated segmental instability (DISI) position. (Fig. 17.1a, b) A magnetic resonance imaging (MRI) study was also reviewed which confirmed a lack of bony union across the fracture site without clear evidence of avascular necrosis. (Fig. 17.2)

Management Options

Numerous surgical options exist for the treatment of pediatric and adolescent scaphoid nonunions, with all of them demonstrating excellent results. Kirschner wire fixation has been shown to be successful [1, 2]; however, more commonly compression screw fixation is now performed if the bone is large enough. [3–5] If bone

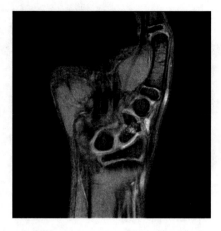

Fig. 17.2 Coronal magnetic resonance imaging (MRI) slices demonstrating the nonunion of the scaphoid waist. Note the lack of bridging bone and signal intensity present about the fracture site. (Courtesy of Shriner's Hospital for Children, Philadelphia, PA)

graft is needed to treat the nonunion, union times are increased by approximately 5 weeks, yet union rates still approach 100%. [1–7] Furthermore, if the distal radial physis is open, distal radial graft should be harvested with great care to avoid physeal bar formation and premature closure of the physis. We prefer instead to use iliac crest in these circumstances. The use of vascularized bone grafting has also been shown to have union rates close to 100%. [8] However, vascularized graft options are limited in the child with open physes. We prefer a modification of the technique described by Fernandez et al [9] that was later published by Tang et al [10] using the superficial volar branch of the radial artery.

Management Chosen

Patients that present with a chronic scaphoid fracture cannot be expected to have the same outcomes as children and adolescents that present with acute fractures and therefore casting is not recommended. Treatment with surgical reduction, bone grafting and compression screw fixation was warranted.

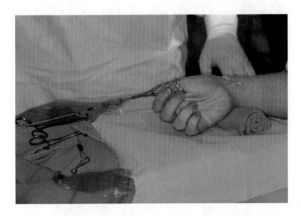

Fig. 17.3 Intraoperative photograph depicting the setup for the treatment of a pediatric scaphoid nonunion including the finger-trap applied traction. (Courtesy of Shriner's Hospital for Children, Philadelphia, PA)

Surgical Technique

The patient was brought to the operating room to undergo fixation of the scaphoid waist nonunion. A nonsterile pneumatic tourniquet was applied to the extremity, and it was then prepped and draped in the usual sterile fashion. Additionally, the ipsilateral iliac crest was prepped and draped in case autologous bone graft was needed. A Carter hand table is used to allow for traction during the procedure. The hand table attaches to a standard operating room table and has a pulley attachment at the end that fits a braided wire with a weight attachment loop on one end and a finger-trap attachment on the other end. This table allows for hands-free, constant dynamic distraction of the fracture site to open up the area of nonunion. (Fig. 17.3) The patient was placed supine and with the arm abducted 90° on the hand table, and 10 pounds of finger-trap traction was applied. A rolled towel was placed under the wrist to create wrist extension.

Initially, the wrist was flexed to permit the lunate to obtain a neutral position. Once the neutral alignment was obtained and confirmed fluoroscopically, the lunate was pinned to the distal radius utilizing a 0.062″ Kirschner wire. A modified Wagner

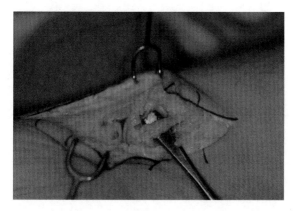

Fig. 17.4 Identification and isolation of the superficial volar branch of the radial artery. (Courtesy of Shriner's Hospital for Children, Philadelphia, PA)

approach was then performed to obtain exposure of the volar scaphoid. In an attempt to augment the vascularity of the proximal fragment, it was decided to perform a vascular pedicle transfer. The superficial volar branch of the radial artery was isolated as it crossed the surgical field. The artery was ligated distally as it entered the thenar muscles and preserved for later use (Fig. 17.4).

Approximately 25 % of the radioscaphocapitate ligament was divided to permit adequate visualization of the fracture site, which demonstrated a 3- to 4-mm gap. The nonunion site was debrided of fibrous tissue and necrotic bone. Excellent punctate bleeding was present from the distal fragment, but only minimal bleeding was present in the proximal fragment. Therefore, it was decided to proceed with autologous bone grafting of the nonunion. The previously dissected vascular pedicle was also placed into the medullary canal of the proximal fragment to augment vascularity to the nonunion site as described above. (Fig. 17.5)

Next, an oblique incision was performed directly over the ipsilateral iliac crest and dissection was carried down to the bone. A piece of tricortical graft was obtained and fashioned to fit in the defect that remained after debridement of the nonunion site. The donor wound was then irrigated and closed in layers, and attention was brought back to the wrist.

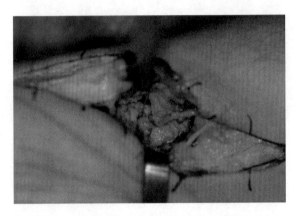

Fig. 17.5 Placement of the superficial volar branch of the radial artery into the proximal fragment medullary canal. (Courtesy of Shriner's Hospital for Children, Philadelphia, PA)

Cancellous bone from the iliac crest was packed around the vascular pedicle, and the tricortical iliac crest was placed in the defect. Once the graft was in position, a headless compression screw was placed across the nonunion site. Excellent alignment and compression were obtained. The Kirschner wire holding the lunate in neutral position was removed, and the traction was released. Lateral fluoroscopic images were obtained, and the lunate was noted to maintain its alignment in a neutral position. Following irrigation and closure of the wound, the patient was placed in a short arm thumb spica cast and awoken from anesthesia.

Clinical Course and Outcome

The patient was maintained in a cast for immobilization until fracture union, which was evident radiographically by 6 weeks postoperatively. (Fig. 17.6) We routinely see union in children at 6 weeks when using the vascular pedicle transfer. Children have

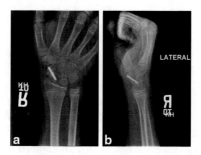

Fig. 17.6 **a** Posteroanterior and **b** lateral views of the wrist demonstrating union of the scaphoid following vascular pedicle transfer, iliac crest bone grafting, and compression screw fixation. (Courtesy of Shriner's Hospital for Children, Philadelphia, PA)

faster times to union than adults, likely due to their increased vascularity and innate ability to heal faster, even in nonunion scenarios. [3] CT scans are not obtained due to concerns of unnecessary radiation in children. At final follow-up of approximately 3 months, the patient no longer had pain and his range of motion was improving.

Clinical Pearls/Pitfalls

- Children have greater healing potential than adults
- The scaphoid is not completely ossified until around 15 years of age, creating the appearance of scapholunate widening which may be misinterpreted as a scapholunate ligament tear
- Vascularized bone grafts from the distal radius are contraindicated in skeletally immature children because of the risk of physeal bar formation
- The superficial volar branch of the radial artery is expendable and reliable, and is sacrificed routinely during the volar approach to the scaphoid

Literature Review and Discussion

Scaphoid fractures are relatively uncommon in the pediatric and adolescent population, representing less than 0.5% of all fractures. [11–13] Furthermore, the vast majority of scaphoid fractures that occur in the pediatric and adolescent population go on to union. [3, 14] Thus, a scaphoid nonunion in a child or adolescent is quite rare, occurring in 1–10% of acute pediatric and adolescent scaphoid fractures. [3, 14] Nonunions of the scaphoid are more likely to occur in this population when the fracture is not initially diagnosed. [15] This may occur due to an unimpressive physical and/or radiographic examination, or due to an inaccurate assessment of the immature carpus on imaging. [6, 16]

Treatment of a pediatric scaphoid nonunion is quite different from that of an acute fracture, as acute fractures that are non-displaced and treated with cast immobilization have a union rate of >90%. However, chronic cases heal with cast immobilization less than 25% of the time. [3, 17–19] Attempts at treatment of chronic scaphoid fractures with casting alone is likely to result in nonunion if the fracture is at the waist or proximal pole, or if the fracture is displaced. [3] Gholson and colleagues reported that chronic fractures are approximately 30 times less likely to achieve union with casting compared to acute fractures. [3] On the contrary, union can be expected to occur in >95% of scaphoid nonunions treated with surgical intervention. [3, 20]

Results following a surgical treatment of scaphoid nonunions demonstrate good-to-excellent range of motion and the absence of pain. [1, 4, 6–8] Surgical complications following the treatment of scaphoid nonunions are extremely rare. [3, 20]

In conclusion, scaphoid nonunions in the pediatric and adolescent populations are quite rare. Prevention is of paramount importance and can occur by prompt and accurate diagnosis and treatment of acute injuries. If a scaphoid nonunion does occur, attempts at treatment with casting should be avoided due to the prolonged periods of immobilization required and a relatively low success rate (less than 25%). Surgical intervention including compression screw fixation, with or without bone grafting, yields excellent outcomes with union rates approaching 100 % and few complications in the pediatric population.

References

1. Maxted MJ, Owen R. Two cases of non-union of carpal scaphoid fractures in children. Injury. 1982;13:441–3.
2. Duteille F, Dautel G. Non-union fractures of the scaphoid and carpal bones in children: surgical treatment. J Pediatr Orthop B. 2004;13:34–8.
3. Gholson JJ, Bae DS, Zurakowski D, Waters PM. Scaphoid fractures in children and adolescents: contemporary injury patterns and factors influencing time to union. J Bone Jt Surg Am. 2011;93:1210–9.
4. Henderson B, Letts M. Operative management of pediatric scaphoid nonunion. J Pediatr Orthop. 2003;23:402–6.
5. Toh S, Miura H, Arai K, Yasumura M, Wada M, Tsubo K. Scaphoid fractures in children: problems and treatment. J Pediatr Orthop. 2003;23:216–21.
6. Mintzer CM, Waters PM. Surgical treatment of pediatric scaphoid fracture nonunions. J Pediatr Orthop. 1999;19:236–9.
7. Southcott R, Rosman MA. Non-union of carpal scaphoid fractures in children. J Bone Jt Surg Br. 1977;59:20–3.
8. Waters PM, Stewart SL. Surgical treatment of nonunion and avascular necrosis of the proximal part of the scaphoid in adolescents. J Bone Jt Surg Am. 2002;84:915–920.
9. Fernandez DL, Eggli S. Non-union of the scaphoid. Revascularization of the proximal pole with implantation of a vascular bundle and bone-grafting. J Bone Jt Surg Am. 1995;77:883–93.
10. Tang P, Fischer CR. A new volar vascularization technique using the superficial palmar branch of the radial artery for the collapsed scaphoid nonunion. Tech Hand Up Extrem Surg. 2010;14:160–72.
11. Mussbichler H. Injuries of the carpal scaphoid in children. Acta Radiol. 1961;53:361–8.
12. Christodoulou AG, Colton CL. Scaphoid fractures in children. J Pediatr Orthop. 1986;6:37–9.
13. Kocher MS, Waters PM, Micheli LJ. Upper extremity injuries in the paediatric athletes. Sports Med. 2000;30:117–35.
14. Fabre O, De Boaeck H, Haentjens P. Fractures and nonunions of the carpal scaphoid in children. Acta Orthop Belg. 2001;67:121–5.
15. Anz AW, Bushnell BD, Bynum DK, Chloros GD, Wiesler ER. Pediatric Scaphoid Fractures. J Am Acad Orthop Surg. 2009;17:77–87.
16. Vahvanen V, Westerlund M. Fracture of the carpal scaphoid in children: a clinical and roentgenological study of 108 cases. Acta Orthop Scand. 1980;51:909–13.

17. Stewart MJ. Fractures of the carpal navicular (scaphoid); a report of 436 cases. J Bone Jt Surg Am. 1954;36:998–1006.
18. Langhoff O, Andersen JL. Consequences of late immobilization of scaphoid fractures. J Hand Surg Br. 1988;13:77–9.
19. Alho A, Kankaanpaa. Management of fractured scaphoid bone. A prospective study of 100 fractures. Acta Orthop Scand. 1975;46:737–43.
20. Masquijo JJ, Willis BR. Scaphoid nonunion in children and adolescents: surgical treatment with bone grafting and internal fixation. J Pediatr Orthop. 2010;30:119–24.

Chapter 18
Partial Scaphoidectomy for Unsalvageable Scaphoid Nonunion

David J. Slutsky

Case Presentation

The patient is a 26-year-old male presenting with a history of a right wrist injury secondary to a skateboard fall 5 years previously. He complained of radial-sided wrist pain at rest that was exacerbated by radial deviation and by wrist extension or with rotation and torque. He was unable to continue working as a roofer due to wrist pain following prolonged use of a hammer or a drill motor. He was also an aspiring professional surfer and travelled internationally for surfing competitions on a regular basis. He experienced minimal improvement following treatment with a thumb spica splint and a radiocarpal corticosteroid injection.

Physical Assessment

On examination of the patient's right hand, there was no thenar wasting. There was 5/5 strength of the abductor pollicus brevis and first dorsal interosseous muscles. Finger range of motion was normal. There was a negative Phalen's test. Two-point discrimi-

David J. Slutsky (✉)
Department of Orthopedics, Harbor-UCLA Medical Center, Torrance, CA, USA
e-mail: d-slutsky@msn.com

© Springer International Publishing Switzerland 2015
J. Yao (ed.), *Scaphoid Fractures and Nonunions,*
DOI 10.1007/978-3-319-18977-2_18

nation was normal at 5 mm. Wrist motion was as follows: flexion 35°, extension 30°, radial deviation 10°, ulnar deviation 20°,
pronation 90°, supination 90°. On examination of the wrist, there
was a mild synovitis in the anatomic snuffbox. On palpation, the
patient experienced tenderness over the scaphoid and radial styloid. He had a positive Watson test.

Diagnostic Studies

Anteroposterior (AP) and lateral X-rays of his right wrist revealed
a hypertrophic nonunion of the distal 1/3 of the scaphoid, along
with radioscaphoid narrowing which was consistent with a scaphoid nonunion advanced collapse scaphoid nonunion advanced
collapse (SNAC) stage 1. There was no evidence of a dorsal intercalated segmental instability (DISI) with a radiolunate angle of
5° (Fig. 18.1a, b). A CT scan revealed hypertrophy of the distal
scaphoid fragment along with cystic change (Fig. 18.2a, b).

Diagnosis

Scaphoid nonunion with radioscaphoid arthrosis (SNAC stage I).

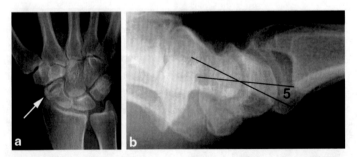

Fig. 18.1 a and **b** AP and lateral view demonstrating a scaphoid nonunion
(arrow) of the distal 1/3 with radioscaphoid narrowing but no DISI deformity. (Published with kind permission of © David J. Slutsky, 2015. All Rights
Reserved)

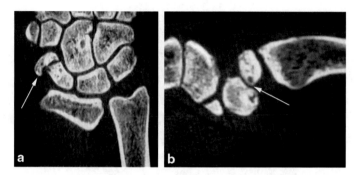

Fig. 18.2 a, b AP and lateral view of a cystic scaphoid nonunion with a hypertrophic distal pole (*arrow*). (Published with kind permission of © David J. Slutsky, 2015. All Rights Reserved)

Management Options

The various management options were discussed with the patient including internal fixation and bone grafting of the scaphoid nonunion ± a limited radial styloidectomy with postoperative immobilization of 3 months or longer versus a distal scaphoid resection and early wrist mobilization.

Management Chosen

The patient did not wish to be immobilized for 3 or more months, mostly due to his competitive surfing schedule, and therefore, elected to proceed with a minimally invasive salvage procedure consisting of an arthroscopic resection of the distal fragment of the scaphoid. He understood that he would likely require a more definitive salvage procedure at some point due to the progression of radiocarpal and midcarpal degenerative joint changes.

The patient was positioned supine under general anesthesia with his arm abducted to 90° under tourniquet control. The thumb was suspended by finger traps from a wrist traction tower with 10 pounds of counter traction. Intraoperative fluoroscopy was employed to assess the adequacy of bone resection and for

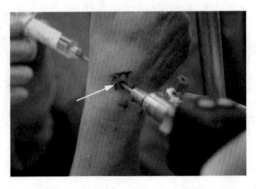

Fig. 18.3 View of the arthoscope inserted in the STT portal (*arrow*). (Published with kind permission of © David J. Slutsky, 2015. All Rights Reserved)

locating the portals as needed. The arthroscopic scaphoidectomy was performed through the midcarpal joint. With the arthroscope introduced in the midcarpal ulnar (MCU) portal, a 2.5-mm shaver was inserted into the midcarpal radial (MCR) portal and used to debride the nonunion site. The scaphotrapeziotrapezoidal ulnar and palmar (STT-U and STT-P) portals are useful for distal 1/3 nonunions. The STT-U portal is located in line with the midshaft axis of the index metacarpal, just ulnar to the extensor pollicus longus (EPL) and radial to the insertion of the extensor carpi radialis tendon into the base of the index metacarpal, at the level of the STT joint (Fig. 18.3). Entry into this portal is facilitated by traction on the index finger. Leaving the EPL to the radial side of the STT-U portal protects the radial artery in the snuffbox from injury. A 2.9-mm and then a 3.5-mm arthroscopic burr were inserted into the MCR or STT-U portal and used to resect the distal scaphoid fragment starting at the nonunion site and moving toward the distal tubercle until the articular surfaces of the trapezoid and trapezium can be seen (Fig. 18.4a, b).

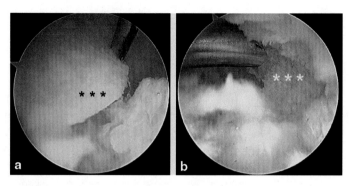

Fig. 18.4 **a** Distal scaphoid fragment at the nonunion site (*) as seen from the MCR portal. **b** Partial resection of the distal fragment with exposed subchondral bone (*). (Published with kind permission of © David J. Slutsky, 2015. All Rights Reserved)

Clinical Course and Outcome

The patient was splinted for 1 week postoperatively then started on a wrist range of motion program, following by progressive strengthening. He returned to competitive surfing at 6th week and unrestricted duty as a carpenter at 8 weeks. At 1-year follow-up, the patient stated that he was able to work as a carpenter with occasional use of a wrist splint. He had no pain at rest, but continued to have mild pain with extremes of radial deviation and wrist extension. On palpation, the patient had mild tenderness over the capitolunate joint but no snuff box tenderness and a negative Watson test. Wrist motion was as follows: flexion 40°, extension 35°, radial deviation 15°, ulnar deviation 20°, pronation 90°, supination 90°. X-rays showed maintenance of a good arthroplasty space with no capitolunate narrowing, but with an increased radiolunate angle of 20°.

Clinical Pearls/Pitfalls

- It is often very difficult to remove the distal scaphoid tuberosity which is still attached to the STT ligaments. Additionally, the distal scaphoid fragment is unstable since it is uncoupled from the proximal scaphoid fragment and tends to be pushed away by the burr.
- A percutaneous 0.62-mm k-wire can be used to hold the distal fragment while it is resected.
- The burr can be placed in the STT-U portal while the scope is in the STT-P portal to resect the distal most part of the scaphoid. The STT-P portal is used to visualize the STT joint and facilitate a resection of the distal scaphoid pole. This portal can be located by inserting a 22-gauge needle just distal to the scaphoid tuberosity while viewing through the STT-U portal.
- Alternatively, the scope can first be placed in the STT-U portal then advanced to the volar capsule to transilluminate the palmar portal site (Fig. 18.5a, b).
- In order to protect the adjacent chondral surfaces, the cancellous bone of the fragment can be resected from the inside while preserving the outer cartilage shell, which can then be removed piecemeal with arthroscopic forceps or a small rongeur by enlarging the portals.

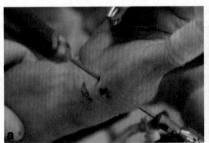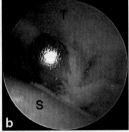

Fig. 18.5 a Intraoperative photo demonstrating the burr in the STT-P portal and the arthroscope in the STT-U portal. **b** View of the burr in the STT-P portal with the arthroscope in the STT-U portal. *T* trapezium, *S* scaphoid. (Published with kind permission of © David J. Slutsky, 2015. All Rights Reserved)

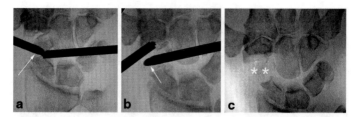

Fig. 18.6 a Fluoroscopy with the scope in the STT-U portal and the burr in the MCR. **b** Following a distal scaphoid resection with the scope in the MCR and the burr in the STT-U portal. **c** Following the resection of the distal scaphoid (*). (Published with kind permission of © David J. Slutsky, 2015. All Rights Reserved)

- Fluoroscopy is used to monitor the completeness of resection (Fig. 18.6a–c).
- An arthroscopic radial styloidectomy can be added if residual impingement is noted.
- If this fails, a small palmar incision can be made to resect the STT ligament and the distal pole can be removed through an enlarged STT-U portal using a rongeur.
- Alternatively, the distal most fragment can be left in place and attached to the STT ligaments as long as there is no radial styloid impingement.
- The burr should be alternated between the MCU, MCR, and STT-U portals to facilitate the resection. A more aggressive shoulder abrader can also be used instead of a burr. A dorsal intercalated instability pattern (DISI) can occur after a distal scaphoid resection and may be a cause of residual wrist pain (Fig. 18.7a, b).

Literature Review and Discussion

Distal scaphoid resection can be regarded as a temporizing procedure for a chronic scaphoid waist or distal pole nonunion. It can relieve pain by alleviating the painful mechanical impingement between the hypertrophic distal pole and the radial styloid. It

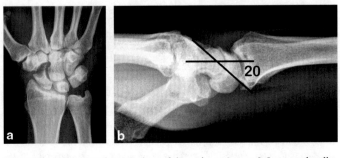

Fig. 18.7 **a** Postoperative AP view of the wrist at 1 year. **b** Increased radio-lunate angle. (Published with kind permission of © David J. Slutsky, 2015. All Rights Reserved)

is especially indicated when the cartilage degeneration and osteophyte formation and deformity are confined mainly to the radial styloid. It enables early wrist motion and does not burn any bridges with regard to more definitive salvage procedures. Advanced degenerative change involving the entire scaphoid fossa or the capitolunate joint are contraindications to this procedure. An intact scapholunate ligament and radioscaphocapitate ligament are prerequisites to the procedure to minimize the risk of a DISI deformity. Because of the increased midcarpal loads following a distal scaphoid resection, the procedure is relatively contraindicated when there is preexisting capitolunate arthritis or if there is a DISI deformity due to the risk of an increased painful subluxation of the capitate [1]. This procedure is not effective as an isolated procedure with a small proximal pole nonunion due to the global carpal instability that occurs following a scaphoidectomy, which mandates a midcarpal fusion. With STT OA, various authors have recommended resecting no more than 4 mm in an attempt to preserve the attachment of the ST ligaments, but this is largely empirical and others have resected the entire distal 1/2 of the scaphoid. There is no comparative study to provide any hard guidelines as to the maximum amount of scaphoid resection. Moritomo et al. [2] however have shown that carpal instability following scaphoid nonunion appears to be related to whether the fracture line passes distal or proximal to the scaphoid apex, where the dorsal intercarpal ligament attaches. Based on this, the author would recommend limiting the resection of the scaphoid distal to the scaphoid apex to limit the risk of developing a postoperative DISI deformity. Malerich et al. [3] proposed the concept of an open distal scaphoid resection arthroplasty procedure in 1999. Ruch et al. [4] reported good pain relief in 3 patients with a chronic scaphoid nonunion associated with avascular necrosis following an arthroscopic resection of the distal scaphoid combined with an arthroscopic radial styloidectomy. His group then reported the outcomes in 13 patients with a persistent nonunion after previous unsuccessful surgical treatment [4]. The authors performed an initial arthroscopic survey to assess the degree of cartilage loss and perform a limited debridement of any partial scapholunate ligament tears. They then performed an open resection of the distal scaphoid pole. Eleven patients achieved complete pain relief while two patients had mild pain only during strenuous activity. The mean wrist flexion improved by 23° and extension increased by 29°. The postoperative DASH score was 25 ± 19 points. There was a significant increase in the radiolunate angle, indicative of a dorsal intercalated segment instability deformity in six patients. Soejima et al. [5] treated 9 patients with an open distal scaphoid resection through a palmar Russe approach (Fig. 18.8a–c) for a chronic scaphoid nonunion. The average patient age was 45.2 years (range, 23–68 years). Seven of the 9 patients had undergone a mean of 2.1 previous failed attempts at bone grafting and internal fixation (range, 1–4 times). The average period from the initial injury to surgery was 94.3

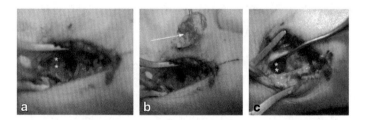

Fig. 18.8 Open distal scaphoid resection. **a** Volar Russe approach demonstrating the nonunited distal scaphoid pole (*). **b** Following resection of the distal scaphoid (*arrow*). **c** Arthroplasty space (*). (Published with kind permission of © David J. Slutsky, 2015. All Rights Reserved)

months (range, 5–372 months). Radiographically, six patients had distal pole radioscaphoid arthritis (SNAC I) and six patients also showed capitolunate arthritis (SNAC III). Preoperatively, seven of the nine patients reported pain with daily use and two patients reported mild pain with light work. At an average follow-up of 28.6 months (range, 12–52 months), 4 patients had no wrist pain and 5 patients had only mild pain with strenuous activity. The composite wrist flexion/extension range of motion improved from 70° (51.4% of the opposite wrist) to 140° (94% of the opposite wrist) and grip strength improved from 18 kg (40% of the opposite wrist) to 30 kg (77% of the opposite wrist). The modified Mayo clinical score improved from 32 ± 16 points before surgery (fair in two patients and poor in seven patients) to 90 ± 7 points after surgery (excellent in six patients and good in three patients) which was statistically significant ($p < 0.0001$). Radiographically, there was no progression of OA in eight patients. Radioscapho-capitate OA developed in one patient with a type II lunate. The radiolunate angle increased from $-26° \pm 12°$ to $-27° \pm 12°$.

In summary, resection of the distal scaphoid pole whether by open or arthroscopic methods is a viable treatment option as a primary palliative procedure for a chronic waist or distal pole scaphoid nonunion that was initially neglected, or after prior failed surgery. The increased capitolunate loads and increased radiolunate angle, however, likely limit the longevity of pain relief following this procedure, which should be thoroughly discussed with the patient.

References

1. Bowers WH, Whipple TL. Arthroscopic anatomy of the wrist. In: McGinty J, Editor. Operative arthroscopy. New York: Raven Press; 1991. pp. 613–23.
2. Malerich MM, Clifford J, Eaton B, Eaton R, Littler JW. Distal scaphoid resection arthroplasty for the treatment of degenerative arthritis secondary to scaphoid nonunion. J Hand Surg Am. 1999;24:1196–205.
3. Ruch DS, Chang DS, Poehling GG. The arthroscopic treatment of avascular necrosis of the proximal pole following scaphoid nonunion. Arthroscopy. 1998;14:747–52.

4. Ruch DS, Papadonikolakis A. Resection of the scaphoid distal pole for symptomatic scaphoid nonunion after failed previous surgical treatment. J Hand Surg Am. 2006;31:588–93.
5. Soejima O, Iida H, Hanamura T, Naito M. Resection of the distal pole of the scaphoid for scaphoid nonunion with radioscaphoid and intercarpal arthritis. J Hand Surg Am. 2003; 28(4):591–6.

Chapter 19
Reconstruction of the Unsalvageable Proximal Pole in Scaphoid Nonunions Utilizing Rib Osteochondral Autograft

Garet Comer and Jeffrey Yao, MD

Case Presentation

The patient was a 19-year-old right-hand-dominant collegiate football lineman who sustained a left scaphoid proximal pole fracture during a game. He was treated with closed reduction and percutaneous fixation with placement of a cannulated headless compression screw (Mini-Acutrak 2, Acumed, Hillsboro, OR). Postoperative radiographs demonstrated maintained reduction and appropriate fixation of the compression screw. Five months after surgery, the patient noted resolution of pain, excellent range of motion, and apparent radiographic union. He was allowed to return to sport, but subsequently reported pain with wrist motion and lifting that limited his functional ability.

J. Yao, MD (✉)
Department of Orthopaedic Surgery, Robert A. Chase Hand and Upper Limb Center, Stanford University Medical Center, Palo Alto, CA, USA
e-mail: jyao@stanford.edu

G. Comer
Robert A. Chase Hand and Upper Limb Center, Stanford University Medical Center, Palo Alto, CA, USA

© Springer International Publishing Switzerland 2015   213
J. Yao (ed.), *Scaphoid Fractures and Nonunions,*
DOI 10.1007/978-3-319-18977-2_19

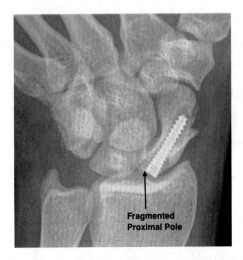

Fig. 19.1 Preoperative X-ray demonstrating lucency around the screw with screw head migration concerning for loss of fixation and proximal pole fragmentation. (Published with kind permission from © Garet Comer and Jeffrey Yao, 2015. All Rights Reserved)

Physical Assessment

Examination of the patient demonstrated tenderness to palpation of the anatomic snuffbox and at the level of the scapholunate interval dorsally. He was not tender at the scaphoid tubercle. Range of motion was mildly diminished with no palpable crepitus.

Diagnostic Studies

Plain radiographs and CT scan were obtained (Figs. 19.1 and 19.2). The plain films demonstrated lucency around the screw with new screw head prominence concerning for loss of fixation with proximal pole fragmentation. The CT scan confirmed nonunion and fragmentation of the proximal pole.

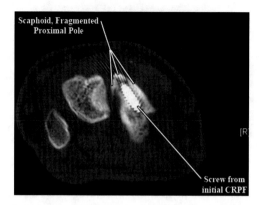

Fig. 19.2 Preoperative axial CT scan confirming proximal pole fragmentation. (Published with kind permission from © Garet Comer and Jeffrey Yao, 2015. All Rights Reserved)

Diagnosis

Based upon the clinical course and imaging findings, this patient was diagnosed with a proximal pole scaphoid nonunion with fragmentation of the proximal pole.

Management Options

The treatment of proximal pole scaphoid nonunions is a challenging problem that does not always yield favorable results. Both vascularized and nonvascularized bone grafting have been advocated for scaphoid nonunions. Iliac–crest bone grafting with compression screw placement is considered a first-line treatment for scaphoid nonunions [1, 2, 3]. However, when avascular necrosis of the proximal pole is present, vascularized bone grafting has demonstrated superior union rates [1, 2]. In a retrospective study reviewing patients with scaphoid nonunions treated with 1,2-inter-compartmental supraretinacular arterial vascularized bone grafting, 18 of 25 patients (72%) with a nonunion at the proximal pole achieved union. However, in those patients with proximal scaphoid nonunion with avascular necrosis, only 8 of 14 (57%) achieved union.

When a proximal pole scaphoid fracture with avascular necrosis leads to fragmentation of the proximal pole, treatment options become more limited. In the rare condition that the fragmented proximal pole is small enough to leave the scapholunate interosseous ligament primarily repairable to the remaining distal scaphoid, the fragment may be excised [4]. However, should excision of a larger proximal pole be necessary, replacement of this necrotic bone should be performed. Interposition of several different materials has been proposed to replace larger proximal pole fragments including silicone implants, fascial interpositions, and pyrocarbon implants. Given complications with silicone synovitis, silicone implants have fallen out of favor [5]. Fascial interposition unfortunately results in loss of scaphoid height and may lead to carpal instability [6]. Pyrocarbon implants have been advocated, but long-term results are still unclear and short-term complications of implant dislocation and need for reoperation have been reported [7].

Other options for replacement of an excised fragmented proximal pole include allograft and autograft reconstruction. Cadaveric scaphoid allografts, though, have the downsides of potential disease transmission, host rejection, and failure of integration [8, 9]. Autograft options include the vascularized medial femoral osteochondral flap and the osteochondral rib autograft. The medial femoral osteochondral flap is a free tissue transfer supplied by periosteal branches of the descending geniculate artery. This flap relies upon the similar contours of the proximal scaphoid and medial femoral trochlear articular surfaces. Early reports demonstrate a high rate of union for this technically demanding procedure [10]. Osteochondral rib autograft is a nonvascularized option that provides a cartilaginous surface to substitute as an articular surface and a bony surface that allows for primary bone healing to the distal pole of the scaphoid.

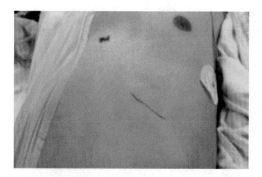

Fig. 19.3 The *left hemithorax* is prepped past the midline, and the incision is marked. (Published with kind permission from © Garet Comer and Jeffrey Yao, 2015. All Rights Reserved)

Management Chosen

This patient was treated with an osteochondral rib autograft. The patient was placed supine on the operating table, and an endotracheal tube was placed after the successful induction of general anesthesia. The patient's operative extremity and his contralateral hemithorax was prepped and draped past the midline (Fig. 19.3). A dorsal approach to the scaphoid was utilized to confirm an unsalvageable proximal pole nonunion, and the distal pole was debrided until bleeding bone was identified. The interspace between the seventh and eighth ribs was identified by palpation, and an incision inferior to and following the interspace was made. The osteochondral junction of the ribs is readily identifiable by a sharply demarcated color change. The seventh rib was circumferentially subperiosteally dissected, elevated off the pleura, and carefully excised (Figs. 19.4 and 19.5). After graft harvest, the wound is flooded with saline and the anesthesiologist delivers a positive inspiration (simulated Valsalva maneuver) to the patient to confirm no air leak. On the back table, the graft is fashioned using a sharp blade to reapproximate the proximal articular surface of the scaphoid while leaving a 2-mm rim of bone to heal to the distal pole (Fig. 19.6). We err on the side of "overstuffing" the graft to help maintain carpal alignment. The graft

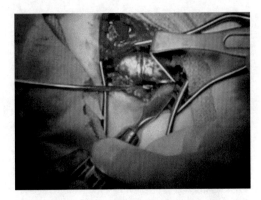

Fig. 19.4 Circumferential subperiosteal elevation of the rib autograft is aided with a Doyen elevator placed deep into the rib to protect the underlying pleura. (Published with kind permission from © Garet Comer and Jeffrey Yao, 2015. All Rights Reserved)

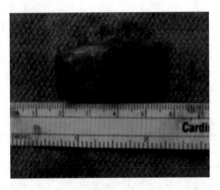

Fig. 19.5 A sharply demarcated color change denotes the osteochondral junction (costal cartilage on the *left* and rib bone on the *right*). (Published with kind permission from © Garet Comer and Jeffrey Yao, 2015. All Rights Reserved)

is inserted and secured with two 0.062 Kirschner wires that are bent and cut at the level of the scaphoid (Fig. 19.7).

Postoperatively the patient was kept immobilized in a thumb spica cast for 10 weeks. Serial X-rays were obtained demonstrating no evidence of fixation failure, and a CT scan was obtained at the 10th week to confirm healing (Fig. 19.8). Once the graft has healed to the distal pole the patient may return to the operating room for pin removal.

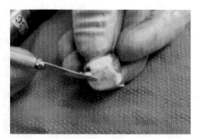

Fig. 19.6 A 69 Beaver blade is useful to whittle the cartilaginous end of the graft to reapproximate the proximal pole's articular surface. (Published with kind permission from © Garet Comer and Jeffrey Yao, 2015. All Rights Reserved)

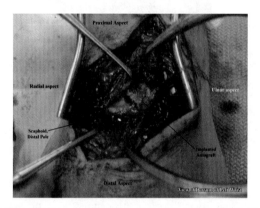

Fig. 19.7 The graft is inserted into the wrist and secured to the distal pole with two 0.062 Kirschner wires bent and cut short. (Published with kind permission from © Garet Comer and Jeffrey Yao, 2015. All Rights Reserved)

Clinical Course and Outcome

The patient tolerated the procedure well and was kept immobilized for 10 weeks postoperatively, after which his pins were removed. At five months, the patient was cleared to return to full activity and resumed training with the football team. He did not play the following season due to the cumulative effect of this injury, a contralateral scaphoid fracture, and a high ankle sprain. However, now 6 years

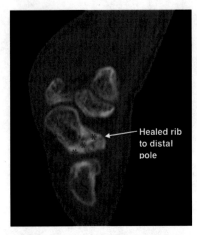

Fig. 19.8 Postoperative sagittal CT scan demonstrating union of the autograft. (Published with kind permission from © Garet Comer and Jeffrey Yao, 2015. All Rights Reserved)

postoperatively, the patient remains very physically active noting no functional limitation and that he regularly performs push-ups without difficulty. The patient notes a palpable defect at the level of seventh rib but no discomfort there. At his final follow-up, his DASH score was 9.1 with a PRWE of 18. Wrist range of motion was as follows. Flexion 65° was compared to 60° on the contralateral side. Extension 70° was compared to 80° on the contralateral side. Radial deviation was 15° compared to 20° on the contralateral side. Ulnar deviation was 40° compared to 40° on the contralateral side. Grip strength was 110 lbs versus 100 lbs on the contralateral side.

Clinical Pearls/Pitfalls

- Watertight periosteal closure is essential to prevent an iatrogenic pneumothorax. To ensure a watertight closure, a red rubber catheter may be threaded through the last remaining opening in the periosteum before the final stitch is tied. The anesthesiologist then provides a forced inspiration as the catheter is simultaneously extracted and the final stitch tied to seal this layer.

- Placing a Doyen elevator around the undersurface of the rib is extremely useful to bluntly dissect the undersurface of the rib free from the parietal pleura (Fig. 19.4).
- When first performing this procedure, it is recommended that a thoracic surgeon be available to help with the dissection, or just in case of any complications.
- Additional cancellous bone graft may be harvested from the medullary canal of the remainder of the rib and impacted into the osteochondral graft.
- A 69 Beaver blade is useful to whittle down the costal cartilage to match the proximal scaphoid articular surface in a fashion analogous to carving a bar of soap (Fig. 19.6).
- The graft should be inserted snuggly in a slightly "overstuffed" manner to restore scaphoid height, reapproximate carpal kinematics, and load the scaphoid to create compression at the graft-recipient interface.
- Proper preoperative patient selection is essential and may be aided by a CT scan to confirm proximal pole fragmentation. Additionally, the rib autograft should not be harvested until visual inspection of the proximal pole confirms that it is nonsalvageable to avoid needless patient morbidity.
- Plain films are difficult to interpret postoperatively and should not be relied upon to confirm union of the autograft. A CT scan should be obtained.

Literature Review and Discussion

To date, three studies have documented the results of proximal scaphoid rib osteochondral autograft in patients with deficiency at the proximal pole. Sandow reported on the results of 47 patients who underwent proximal scaphoid rib osteochondral replacement at a median follow-up of 15 months [9]. All patients noted better wrist function postoperatively with an average modified Green and O'Brien Wrist Function Score of 65 (out of 100) preoperatively and 85 at final follow-up. None of the 47 patients required a subsequent wrist arthrodesis or salvage procedure.

Similarly, Veitch and colleagues noted that 13 of 14 patients treated with a rib osteochondral autograph experienced improvement in wrist function with improved grip strength, less pain, and maintenance of wrist motion [8]. The mean preoperative Green and O'Brien Wrist Function Score of 54 improved to 79 at a mean of 64 months postoperatively.

We have reported on three young, active patients at our institution that underwent this procedure for nonsalvageable proximal pole scaphoid nonunions [11]. At a mean follow-up of 58 months, the average Quick DASH score was 12.

None of the patients in these three series developed nonunion, deterioration of carpal alignment, donor site complications, or other major complications. Fortunately, the incidence of encountering a nonsalvageable proximal pole of the scaphoid is quite low. However, when it occurs, it is beneficial to be familiar with procedures such as this to potentially treat the patient rather than resorting to a salvage procedure.

References

1. Merrell GA, Wolfe SW, Slade JF 3rd. Treatment of scaphoid non-unions: quantitative meta-analysis of the literature. J Hand Surg Am. 2002;27:685–91.
2. Waitayawinyu T, Pfaeffle HJ, McCallister WV, Nemechek NM, Trumble TE. Management of scaphoid nonunions. Orthop Clin North Am. 2007;38:237–49, vii.
3. Krimmer H, Kremling E, van Schoonhoven J, Prommersberger KJ, Hahn P. Proximal scaphoid pseudarthrosis—reconstruction by dorsal bone screw and spongiosa transplantation. Handchir Mikrochir Plast Chir. 1999;31:174–7.
4. Garcia-Elias M, Lluch A. Partial excision of scaphoid: is it ever indicated? Hand Clin. 2001;17:687–95.
5. Haussman P. Long-term results after silicone prosthesis replacement of the proximal pole of the scaphoid bone in advanced scaphoid nonunion. J Hand Surg Br. 2002;27:417–23.

6. Eaton RG, Akelman E, Eaton BH. Fascial implant arthroplasty for treatment of radioscaphoid degenerative disease. J Hand Surg Am. 1989;14:766–74.
7. Gras M, Wahegaonkar, A, Mathoulin, C. Treatment of avascular necrosis of the proximal pole of the scaphoid by arthroscopic resection and prosthetic semireplacement arthroplasty using the pyrocabon adaptive proximal scaphoid implant (APSI): long-term functional outcomes. J Wrist Surg. 2012;1(2):159–64.
8. Veitch S, Blake SM, David H. Proximal scaphoid rib graft arthroplasty. J Bone Joint Surg Br. 2007;89:196–201.
9. Sandow MJ. Costo-osteochondral grafts in the wrist. Tech Hand Up Extrem Surg. 2001;5:165–72.
10. Bürger HK, Windhofer C, Gaggi AJ, Higgins JP. Vascularized medial femoral trochlea osteocartilaginous flap reconstruction of proximal pole scaphoid nonunions. J Hand Surg Am. 2013;38(4):690–700.
11. Yao J, Read B, Hentz VR. The fragmented proximal pole scaphoid nonunion treated with rib autograft: case series and review of the literature. J Hand Surg Am. 2013;38(11):2188–92.

Chapter 20
Recalcitrant Proximal Pole Nonunions Reconstructed with Medial Femoral Condyle Osteoarticular Graft

James P. Higgins

Case Presentation

A 27-year-old right-hand dominant male presented to the office with pain in the anatomic snuffbox and limitation in the range of motion and grip strength of the right hand. The patient was identified as having a proximal pole scaphoid fracture 2.5 years prior to presentation. He initially underwent 8 weeks of casting at the time of injury and was thought to have healed his fracture. Fourteen months later, he was found to have a nonunited fracture and underwent 1,2 intracompartmental supraretinacular pedicled vascularized bone grafting from the distal radius via a dorsal approach and screw fixation.

Six months later, CT scan images demonstrated a persistent nonunion with cystic changes at the nonunion site. The patient was referred for the revision treatment of the scaphoid nonunion or salvage procedures.

J. P. Higgins (✉)
Curtis National Hand Center, MedStar Union Memorial Hospital,
Baltimore, MD, USA
e-mail: jameshiggins10@hotmail.com

© Springer International Publishing Switzerland 2015   225
J. Yao (ed.), *Scaphoid Fractures and Nonunions,*
DOI 10.1007/978-3-319-18977-2_20

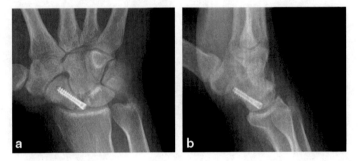

Fig. 20.1 a and **b** Preoperative anteroposterior and lateral radiographs. (Published with kind permission of © James Higgins, 2015. All Rights Reserved.)

Physical Assessment

On examination, the patient demonstrated a well-healed scar on the dorsal aspect of his wrist. He had full digital range of motion. His wrist extension was limited to 30°, flexion to 20°, ulnar deviation to 25°, and radial deviation to 0°. He demonstrated full forearm pronosupination. His grip strength was diminished as compared to his contralateral uninvolved side.

Diagnostic Studies

X-rays demonstrated a dorsal headless bone screw traversing a very small proximal pole nonunion fragment. The nonunion site exhibited cystic formation and bone loss. There was no evidence of arthritic changes in the radial carpal or midcarpal joint. (Fig. 20.1)

CT scan images demonstrated with greater clarity the small dimensions of the small proximal pole segment and a humpback flexion deformity at the nonunion site (Fig. 20.2). The lunate is positioned in a neutral posture.

Diagnosis

Recalcitrant proximal pole scaphoid nonunion following failure of a previous vascularized bone graft procedure from the distal radius.

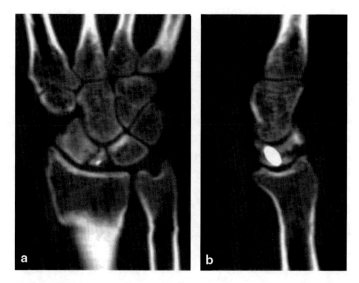

Fig. 20.2 a and **b** Preoperative coronal and sagittal CT scans revealing a small proximal pole fragment and humpback deformity. (Published with kind permission of © James Higgins, 2015. All Rights Reserved.)

Management Options

Given the failure of a previous well-performed treatment with a vascularized distal radius bone graft, revision vascularized bone grafting from the radius does not offer any advantages in achieving scaphoid healing. The very small proximal pole fragment presents a particular challenge in achieving fixation with subsequent nonunion surgery particularly given the osseous changes from the previous screw fixation.

Options for reconstruction of the scaphoid include revision ORIF with a vascularized corticocancellous bone flap from another site such as the medial femoral condyle (MFC), or proximal pole excision and replacement with vascularized osteochondral reconstruction from the medial femoral trochlea (MFT). Options for salvage procedures would include scaphoid excision and midcarpal fusion or proximal row carpectomy.

Management Chosen

Due to the patient's young age and lack of arthritic changes, the patient was deemed a candidate for revision ORIF of the scaphoid nonunion. Because of the failure of previous vascularized cortico-cancellous grafting, the small size of the proximal pole fragment, and the poor quality of the proximal pole fragment after previous screw fixation, the patient was felt to be an ideal candidate for proximal pole scaphoid excision and medial femoral trochlea vascularized osteochondral reconstruction.

Surgical Technique

The MFT osteochondral flap, provides a convex cartilaginous segment of bone with an arc of curvature very similar to that of the greater curvature of the proximal scaphoid. A segment of osteochondral bone is harvested in continuity with the transverse branch of the descending geniculate artery. The source vessel is the same as the conventional MFC corticoperiosteal flap (Fig. 20.3). However, the MFT's terminal branch (transverse branch) is distinct from the longitudinal branch typically used for the MFC flap. The osteochondral segment is harvested to mimic the deficit created after resection of the proximal pole fragment and additional portions of the proximal scaphoid beyond the nonunion site (Fig. 20.4).

This resection of additional scaphoid distal to the nonunion site converts the proximal pole nonunion conceptually into a waist-level osteosynthesis site. During resection of the proximal scaphoid, cartilage on the lesser curvature that articulates with the midcarpal joint is preserved. Additionally, the distal-most segments of the dorsal and volar scapholunate interosseous ligament are likewise preserved if possible. Preservation of the thin cartilage layer and distal scapholunate ligament is facilitated by maintaining the capsular integrity of the midcarpal joint. The resection is completed with the goal of opening only the radicarpal joint. The only cartilage-bearing surface of the medial femoral trochlea flap is oriented to articulate solely with the scaphoid fossa of the radius (Fig. 20.5).

The flap is inserted such that the vascular pedicle and periosteum are oriented dorsal in the wrist (Fig. 20.6). The pedicle is

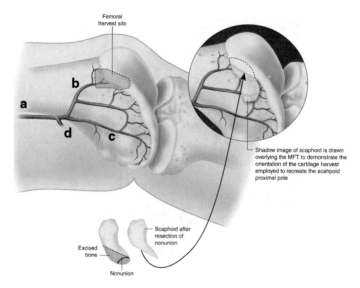

Fig. 20.3 Diagram of the vascular tree of the descending geniculate artery. Note the course of the transverse branch and its relationship to the proximal trochlea. Also demonstrated is the area of typical harvest and its orientation in the reconstructed scaphoid. (Published with kind permission of © The Curtis National Hand Center. All Rights Reserved.)

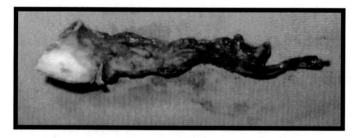

Fig. 20.4 The harvested osteochondral graft with pedicle. (Published with kind permission of © James Higgins, 2015. All Rights Reserved.)

draped in a distal direction and is gently routed into the snuffbox for microvascular anastomosis end-to-side into the radial artery and associated veins.

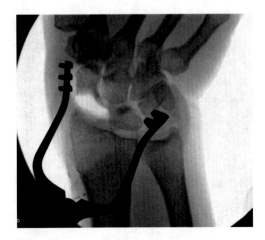

Fig. 20.5 Intraoperative fluoroscopic view of the scaphoid after generous resection of the nonunion fragment and an additional portion of native scaphoid distal to the nonunion site. Note the preservation of the convex cartilage segment that articulates with the midcarpal joint. By preparing the scaphoid resection in this manner, the proximal pole nonunion is converted to a less-challenging waist-level osteosynthesis site. Additionally, this preparation allows the only cartilage-bearing surface of the MFT osteochondral segment to articulate with the scaphoid fossa, while preserved native scaphoid cartilage articulates with the midcarpal joint. (Published with kind permission of © James Higgins, 2015. All Rights Reserved.)

The conversion of a poor-quality small proximal pole nonunion fragment to a considerably larger dense osteochondral flap greatly facilitates fixation. Headless cannulated screw fixation is directed through the cartilage surface of the flap across the waist-level osteosynthesis site and into the distal pole. This screw is often directed in a more longitudinal orientation than conventional scaphoid screw placement in order to achieve a good interface with the distal pole bone fragment and avoid the pathway of the previously failed screw fixation.

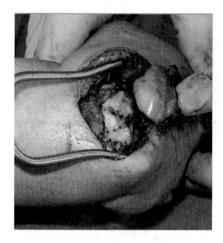

Fig. 20.6 Sizing the graft compared to the native scaphoid. The pedicle is draped into the anatomic snuffbox. (Published with kind permission of © James Higgins, 2015. All Rights Reserved.)

Clinical Course and Outcome

The patient demonstrated a healed scaphoid reconstruction confirmed with CT scan obtained 12 weeks after surgery. He achieved complete resolution of pain and tenderness. His digital range of motion and pronosupination remained full. His wrist extension in 12 weeks was 35°, flexion was 55°, ulnar deviation was 25°, and radial deviation was 5°.

Postoperative knee discomfort created a gait disturbance for approximately 6 weeks. No immobilization or gait assistance (i.e., crutch, cane) were required. Twelve weeks after surgery, his knee became pain-free with full range of motion. He was able to participate in his routine athletic endeavors which include running, soccer, and biking. Follow-up radiographs 1 year after the surgery demonstrated no development of arthritic changes and a well preserved and normal SL angle and interval. (Fig. 20.7)

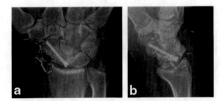

Fig. 20.7 a and **b** Postoperative AP and lateral radiographs 1 year after reconstruction. (Published with kind permission of © James Higgins, 2015. All Rights Reserved.)

Clinical Pearls/Pitfalls

- A segment of osteochondral bone is harvested in continuity with the transverse branch of the descending geniculate artery.
- The osteochondral segment is harvested to mimic the deficit created after resection of the proximal pole fragment and additional portions of the proximal scaphoid beyond the nonunion site.
- Resection of additional scaphoid distal to the nonunion site converts the proximal pole nonunion conceptually into a waist-level osteosynthesis site.
- Preservation of the thin cartilage layer and distal scapholunate ligament is facilitated by maintaining the capsular integrity of the midcarpal joint.
- The screw is often directed in a more longitudinal orientation than conventional scaphoid screw placement to achieve a good interface with the distal pole bone fragment and avoid the pathway of the previously failed screw fixation.

Literature Review and Discussion

The descending genicular artery system has demonstrated value as a donor for microvascular reconstruction. In upper extremity surgery, it has been shown to be of use as a pliable corticoperiosteal flap, a corticocancellous semi-structural flap, and a skin-bearing flap. Its transverse branch has been well studied and demonstrated to supply a periosteal filigree of vessels to the cartilage-bearing area of the proximal aspect of the medial trochlea of the patellofemoral joint. This convex surface has been demonstrated to be of similar contour to the greater curvature of the scaphoid as well as the mirror–image scaphoid fossa.

These qualities have made the MFT flap a useful tool in treating recalcitrant proximal pole scaphoid nonunions. The sole series reporting its use reported on 16 patients with a minimum of 6-month follow-up (average follow-up was 14 months with a range from 6 to 72 months) [1]. The median age of the patients was 30 years with the range of 18–47. The average number of previous operations was 1 with the range of 0–3. Seven of 16 patients were smokers. The authors reported healed scaphoid reconstructions confirmed by CT scan in 15/16 patients. In one patient, healing was not achieved and the patient is considering salvage operations. Most (12 of 16) patients reported complete pain relief while 4 of 16 reported improvement without complete pain relief. Pronosupination and digital range of motion were unaffected when comparing preoperative to postoperative values. Preoperative extension averaged 45.7° and postoperative extension averaged 46°. Preoperative flexion averaged 43° and postoperative flexion averaged 43.8°. Radiographically the analysis of the intercarpal relationships demonstrated relatively unchanged scapholunate angles with an average of 51.6° preoperatively and 48.6° postoperatively.

MFT scaphoid reconstruction is indicated in young patients with scaphoid nonunions demonstrating a very small proximal pole fracture fragment that has failed previous attempts of reconstruction, or less commonly, in young patients with extremely small proximal scaphoid nonunion without prior surgeries. In these situations, conventional reconstructive techniques, likely, will not provide both improved vascularity and rigid internal fixation. When the proximal fragment is extremely small and particularly when it has been previously damaged by single or multiple attempts at screw fixation, it is difficult to achieve adequate fixation. Conventional vascularized or nonvascularized correction procedures require preservation of this small damaged cartilage shell. Often, however, this shell is unsalvageable. The medial femoral trochlea flap provides the surgeon the ability to widely resect this damaged fragment and resect distally into the normal scaphoid fragment enlarging the nonunion site and converting the proximal pole fracture to a waist level defect. This larger defect can be filled because of the ability to transfer this morphologically similar convex osteocartilaginous flap. The larger size of the flap enables the surgeon to easily achieve rigid internal fixation on both proximal and distal fragments. These attributes enable the surgeon to deliver both improved vascularity and fixation to difficult nonunion cases and achieve union despite previous failures. It also enables the surgeon to make a challenging technical case somewhat more feasible by supplying fixation and not feeling compelled to preserve a damaged and compromised proximal cartilaginous shell.

In order to maintain intercarpal relationships after resecting the majority of the scapholunate ligament and proximal pole, additional care is required. The distal-most cartilaginous shell of the native scaphoid that effaces the midcarpal joint as well as the distal-most aspects of the dorsal scapholunate ligament is preserved if possible. In addition to the stability afforded by the distal scapholunate ligament segment, biomechanical evidence has demonstrated that the replacement of the resected proximal pole (often with bone loss and humpback deformity) with a larger osteochondral graft may provide correction of scapholunate alignment, even in the absence of primary and secondary soft tissue stabilizers [2]. These data would suggest that oversized osteochondral flaps ("scaphoid overstuffing") may permit complete resection of the proximal pole segment and scapholunate ligament in these difficult cases without resultant rotary subluxation of the scaphoid.

A concern with osteochondral flap harvest is that of donor site morbidity. These patients will typically report transient discomfort in the knee after medial femoral trochlea harvest for approximately 3 months. Thereafter, they are routinely able to return to normal ambulation as well as sporting activities without difficulty.

While these findings are quite promising for addressing this very difficult problem of recalcitrant proximal pole scaphoid nonunions, there are many unaddressed questions. Long-term radiographic and subjective outcomes are needed to determine the value of this reconstructive option and its ability to preserve function and avoid arthritic changes. Further basic research is also warranted on determining the relative value of periosteal and subchondral vascular supply to cartilage in relation to that of synovial perfusion.

References

1. Bürger HK, Windhofer C, Gaggl AJ, Higgins JP. Vascularized medial femoral trochlea osteocartilaginous flap reconstruction of proximal pole scaphoid nonunions. J Hand Surg Am. 2013;38(4):690–700.
2. Capito AE, Higgins JP. Scaphoid overstuffing: the effects of the dimensions of scaphoid reconstruction on scapholunate alignment. J Hand Surg Am. 2013;38(12):2419–25.

Suggested Readings

Higgins JP, Burger HK. Proximal scaphoid arthroplasty using the medial femoral trochlea flap. J Wrist Surg. 2013;02(03):228–33.

Higgins JP, Burger HK. Osteochondral flaps from the distal femur: expanding applications, harvest sites, and indications. J Reconstr Microsurg. 2014;30:483–490.

Iorio ML, Masden DL, Higgins JP. Cutaneous angiosome territory of the medial femoral condyle osteocutaneous flap. J Hand Surg. 2012;37(5):1033–41.J. P. Higgins

Chapter 21
Unsalvageable Scaphoid Nonunion: Implant Arthroplasty

Marco Rizzo, Alessio Pedrazzini and Maurizio Corradi

Case Presentation

A 34-year-old right hand dominant male, manual laborer presented with pain and swelling over the dorsal radial aspect of his right wrist. He fell onto his outstretched hand approximately 4 years prior to presentation while at work and considered his injury to be a "sprain." He initially recovered and returned to work without restriction. However, 6 months prior to presentation, he developed progressive pain, swelling, and weakness.

Physical Assessment

The physical exam demonstrated limited range-of-motion with flexion–extension of 40° and 30°, respectively. In addition, he had limited radial–ulnar deviation of 5° and 15°, respectively. He had full and symmetric forearm pronation–supination. He had significant weakness compared to his contralateral side (16 vs. 50 kg grip

M. Rizzo (✉)
Department of Orthopedic Surgery, Mayo Clinic, Rochester, MN, USA
e-mail: Rizzo.marco@mayo.edu

A. Pedrazzini
Department of Orthopaedic Surgery and Traumatology, Oglio Po Hospital, Cremona, Italy

M. Corradi
Department of Orthopedic and Hand Surgery, Hospital University of Parma, Parma, Italy

The original version of this chapter was revised. An erratum can be found at
https://doi.org/10.1007/978-3-319-18977-2_28

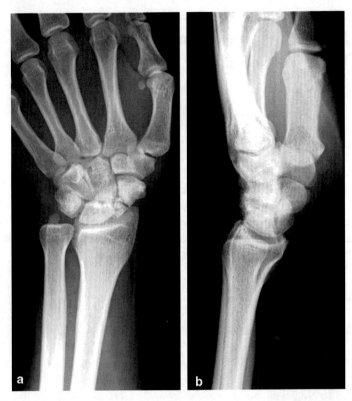

Fig. 21.1 **a** Anteroposterior and **b** lateral radiographs of the patient demonstrate long-standing nonunion of the scaphoid with proximal pole sclerosis. (Published with kind permission of © Alessio Pedrazzini, 2015. All rights reserved)

strength). In addition to swelling over the dorsal–radial aspect of the wrist, palpation of the snuffbox generated significant pain.

Diagnostic Studies and Diagnosis

Anteroposterior and lateral radiographs (Fig. 21.1) demonstrated a scaphoid nonunion with cystic changes, suspicion for avascularity of the proximal pole and collapse which was confirmed with

Fig. 21.2 Coronal CT scan better illustrates the cystic changes at the nonunion site. (Published with kind permission of © Alessio Pedrazzini, 2015. All rights reserved)

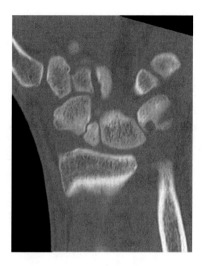

computed tomography (CT) scan (Fig. 21.2). The sclerosis and cystic changes suggested that salvage of the proximal pole of the scaphoid was considered to be challenging and unlikely to be successful.

Management Options

Surgical treatment options for this difficult problem are variable and can be quite challenging. As previously mentioned, while vascularized bone grafting may be attempted, it is not likely to be successful in such a chronic nonunion and in the setting of avascular necrosis. Additional options include partial scaphoid excision with and without soft-tissue interposition, scaphoidectomy and four-corner fusion, proximal row carpectomy, and proximal or complete scaphoid arthroplasty.

Fig. 21.3 The pyrocarbon
implant (APSI). (Published
with kind permission of ©
Alessio Pedrazzini, 2015.
All rights reserved)

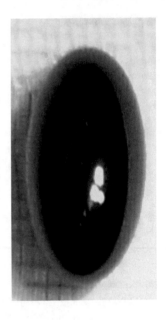

Management Chosen

Given the absence of degenerative changes in the radiocarpal joint
and the well-maintained overall carpal alignment, this patient was
deemed a candidate for partial scaphoid replacement. The patient
underwent proximal pole scaphoid arthroplasty. For this case, the
adaptive proximal scaphoid implant (APSI; Tournier, Montbon-
not Saint Martin, France) was utilized (Fig. 21.3). The implant is
made of biologically inert pyrolytic carbon and has favorable wear
characteristics. Its elastic modulus is similar to cortical bone, and
animal studies have shown that it is biologically friendly to cartilage and bone. In addition, it is much stronger and more durable
than silicone allowing for maintenance of carpal height and carpal alignment. Indications for proximal pole arthroplasty include
an unsalvageable scaphoid, avascular necrosis, and collapse. The
ideal patient would also have no evidence of arthritic changes in
the scaphoid fossa of the radius and generally well maintained or
minimal loss of carpal alignment.

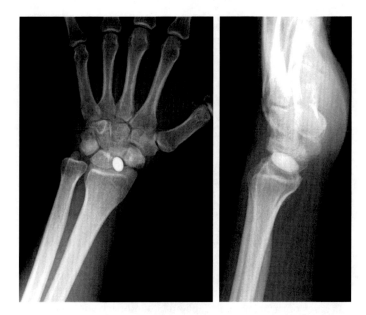

Fig. 21.4 a Anteroposterior and **b** lateral radiographs 2 years following surgery. Note the maintenance of carpal alignment and stability of the implant position. (Published with kind permission of © Alessio Pedrazzini, 2015. All rights reserved)

Clinical Course and Outcome

The patient had excellent pain relief and improved strength and motion following surgery. Postoperative radiographs at 2 years following surgery are shown in Fig. 21.4. In addition to maintaining stable position, the carpal alignment was restored. He had no snuffbox pain. His grip strength improved to 35 kg, and the range-of-motion demonstrated a flexion–extension of 40° and 40° and radial–ulnar deviation of 10° and 25°, respectively. He was able to return to his employment without restriction.

Clinical Pearls/Pitfalls

Pearls

- A small dorsal open incision or arthroscopic approach can be utilized for proximal pole excision.
- Excision of the proximal pole is facilitated by release of the scapholunate ligament.
- The proximal pole is removed using a forceps or hemostat.
- Use of fluoroscopy is helpful in confirming the resection and examining the position of the implant.
- Implant size is based on the excised proximal pole and radiographs.
- Trialing can help confirm stability and optimize for the right sized implant.
- While early motion can be initiated after 1 week, casting for 2–3 weeks may afford greater stability.
- In cases of early (stage 1 scaphoid nonunion advanced collapse) arthritis, a radial styloidectomy may also be performed.

Pitfalls

- Care should be taken to avoid neurovascular and extensor tendon injury during the approach and scaphoid proximal pole excision.
- Overly aggressive volar capsule of the wrist and radioscapholunate ligament release during excision of the scaphoid may cause instability and ulnar translation of the carpus.
- Instability can occur with premature motion, and the patient should work toward activity as tolerated through 6 weeks following surgery.

Literature Review and Discussion

Unsalvageable scaphoid nonunions with proximal pole avascular necrosis, sclerosis, and collapse pose a significant challenge for hand surgeons. Distal or proximal pole excision has been described in the past [1–4]. It is a relatively simple solution and straightforward rehabilitation for this difficult problem. Some investigators have reported encouraging early-term outcomes with this technique [2, 3]. However, problems with carpal malalignment and maintenance of carpal height resulting in recurrent pain and progression of arthritis may be a problem [2, 5, 6].

Partial and complete excision of the scaphoid with implant or soft-tissue arthroplasty has also been described for the unsalvageable scaphoid nonunion [7–16]. Complete scaphoid replacements include both silicone and metal materials. Inspired by A.T. Moore's outcomes with hip hemiarthroplasty, a vitallium scaphoid arthroplasty was introduced in the 1940s [13, 17, 18]. While Legge [18] reported good outcomes in seven cases, Waugh and Reuling [17] felt that the results were too preliminary to make any conclusions in the three patients they treated. Leslie et al. reported a 43-year follow-up on a patient who underwent treatment with a vitallium scaphoid for unsalvageable nonunion [13]. While the implant remained quite stable radiographically and the patient had a functional range-of-motion, they also observed that the patient had pain and X-rays demonstrated significant erosion of the implant into the radius. Acrylic scaphoid replacements were introduced a short time later [19]. Like vitallium, preliminary outcomes were encouraging. Agerholm and Lee shared their experience with the acrylic scaphoid arthroplasty in a review of 16 patients followed between 1 and 8 years [20]. Despite the presence of pain in all but four cases, satisfactory motion, grip, and function were achieved in 14 of 16 wrists. While carpal collapse was present in five patients following surgery, it developed in only three cases compared to preoperative radiographs. Osteoarthritis was noted and graded as marked in five wrists, slight in six wrists, and absent in three. Two patients ultimately required implant removal. Agner published his experience with an acrylic silicone arthroplasty for scaphoid nonunion in seven cases with a 9- to 11-year follow-up [21]. Early improvement in range-of-motion was obtained in all cases. However, four patients were unable to return to work secondary to pain and another, despite early encouraging results, developed pain at 1 year following surgery. These five patients required removal of the implant. One of the two patients whose implant remained had radiographic evidence of severe arthritis 10 years following surgery with considerable pain. With only one case achieving a satisfactory outcome, the author was displeased with his experience.

Silicone scaphoid arthroplasty was introduced in the 1960s [22]. The premise of its use was in part secondary to the success with small-joint arthroplasty. The hope was that it would function more as a spacer and its material properties would minimize the progression of arthritis, yet be strong enough to maintain carpal alignment. Despite some encouraging preliminary reports, outcomes with silicone replacement for nonunion and scaphoid diseases have been generally poor [23–25]. Kleinert et al. published their experience with 33 patients who underwent treatment with silicone arthroplasty for the scaphoid with a 3-year average follow-up period [24]. Motion only improved slightly, and grip strength did not improve. Unfortunately, 13 (of 23 patients available for follow-up) went on to develop carpal collapse, and 9 of them had obvious subluxation of the spacer. Thirteen additional surgeries in ten patients were required. Smith et al. introduced us to the concerns associated with silicone synovitis with the carpal silicone implants [25]. A long-term clinical and radiographic analysis performed by Carter et al. demonstrated that 75 % of patients developed osseous changes and over half had significant pain associated with this problem [23].

As a result of complications associated with silicone, Swanson introduced a titanium scaphoid implant in the 1980s [16]. In their report, the authors outlined the indications and technique and shared their experience with 102 implants, among which 78 patients (85 wrists) were available for follow-up of an average 5.7 years. Forty-one of these were treated for scaphoid nonunion. Results demonstrated 97 % were extremely satisfied. Two developed arthritis and were revised to arthrodesis. One had persistent pain. The average wrist flexion–extension was 36° and 33°, respectively. Radial–ulnar deviation was 10° and 24°, respectively. Grip strength improved

40 % on average. Radiographs demonstrated that carpal alignment was well maintained and there were no significant osseous changes or problems related to the titanium alloy. Sixty-nine patients were able to return to pre-injury work activities. Spingardi and Rosello published their experience with the use of titanium scaphoid arthroplasty as well [15]. The authors examined 112 cases performed over a 15-year period, and they detailed the indications and their preferred technique along with outcomes. Seventy-five patients were available for follow-up analysis at an average 46-month follow-up interval. Clinical outcomes demonstrated nearly 75 % of patients had improved or functional flexion–extension arc of motion and the average grip strength was 80 % of contralateral side. 85 % of patients had no pain, 8 % had mild pain and 7 % had pain with activity, and all patients were able to return to their previous employment. Fifty-six (of 75) patients were considered to have a satisfactory or excellent result. The authors concluded that titanium scaphoid arthroplasty for unsalvageable nonunion, in the absence of arthritic changes, is a valid alternative to other salvage procedures.

Partial arthroplasty is an alternative to complete scaphoid excision and replacement. With less bone resection, structural stability may be preserved and less loading on the implant may minimize wear and improve survivorship. This concept was proposed by Bentzon and Randlov-Madsen in 1945 [26]. In their report of soft-tissue interposition at the nonunion site, they had three cases of small proximal pole fractures that underwent excision and interposition. They felt that those cases did particularly well. Qvick and Wilhelm described a tendon interposition arthroplasty following partial scaphoid resection and felt that the results were quite good [27]. Pain relief was predictable and most patients had improved function, despite slight reduction in motion and diminishment of strength. The authors also lauded their minimal complication rate and favorable rehabilitation needs.

Silicone replacement of the proximal pole has also been proposed as an alternative to complete replacement. Egloff et al. reported on long-term (13-year average) outcomes with silicone lunate and scaphoid arthroplasties in 39 wrists [10]. Sixteen had complete replacement of the scaphoid, while nine had partial scaphoid replacement. Clinical results were stratified into excellent, satisfactory, and poor. The partial replacement group had 41% excellent, 41% satisfactory, and 18% poor outcomes; the total replacement group had 23% excellent, 49% satisfactory, and 28% poor outcomes. Unfortunately, silicone synovitis was observed in all cases, and the authors concluded that they no longer recommend replacement for the scaphoid or lunate bones. Hausman also examined outcomes of 11 patients treated with proximal pole scaphoid excision and silicone arthroplasty treated between 1980 and 1984 [12]. Two patients had reoperations: one underwent excision for dislocation and another had arthrodesis for pain 5 years following surgery. The nine remaining patients were followed for an average 14 years. Despite good clinical results in most cases, the author noted significant silicone synovitis, carpal collapse, and progression of arthritis over time. For these reasons, he concluded that this procedure was abandoned.

The pyrolytic carbon implant is a carbon-matrix implant that is made by machining a graphite substrate at high temperatures in a carbon gas-heated chamber. The implant has some theoretical material advantages over metal and silicone prostheses. Its elastic modulus is similar to that of cortical bone, and it has excellent wear characteristics. In addition, it is biologically inert and its polished surface has been shown to compare favorably to materials such as cobalt chrome and titanium [28]. One additional possible advantage over other implants is that pyrocarbon may be suitable in patients who have already begun to have evidence of scaphoid nonunion advanced collapse (SNAC). These features suggest that it may be suitable as a spacer and it has been utilized as a proximal pole scaphoid replacement [9, 11, 14, 29]. This first published experience with the pyrocarbon proximal pole arthroplasty was published in 2000 by Pequignot et al. [14]. At an average 6-year follow-up period, 25 cases (14 of scaphoid nonunion/SNAC, 10 of scapholunate advanced collapse (SLAC), and 1 failed silicone arthroplasty) were included in this retrospective review. Postoperatively, an 88% satisfaction rate was noted with improvement of strength and maintenance of functional arc of motion. Pain resolved completely in 60% of patients, and seven patients described pain that persisted with activity. All patients were able to return to their prior work. Radiolunate angle improved in 6 cases, remained unchanged in 15, and worsened in 4. Carpal height was maintained in all cases. Poorer results were found in patients with greater carpal instability preoperatively. Daruwalla et al. prospectively analyzed 12 patients treated with the APSI proximal scaphoid treated over a 3-year period [9]. No complications were noted and all patients expressed satisfaction in this early-term analysis of an average 18-month follow-up. Pain, range-of-motion, and grip/pinch strengths all fared favorably. In addition, all patients were able to return to work, and disability of arm, hand, and shoulder (DASH) scores were excellent. Radiographic analysis demonstrated maintenance of carpal alignment. The authors concluded that while longer-term results are necessary to better validate their use, pyrocarbon implant arthroplasty for unsalvageable scaphoid nonunion has promise. Gras et al. published a retrospective longer-term outcomes in a multicenter cohort treated with arthroscopic resection of the proximal pole and interposition of the APSI, at an average 5-year follow-up interval [11]. The study included 14 patients with a mean 8.7-year follow-up period. Pain improved from preoperative Visual-Analog Scale (VAS) pain scores of 7.5 to 0.7. Extension improved from 45 to 60°; flexion improved from 32 to 53 following surgery. Grip strength also improved from 15.8 to 34.6 kg. The authors experienced three complications which included two cases of implant subluxation (one treated with surgical correction and another graduated to a partial wrist fusion). Another case required subsequent radial styloidectomy. They concluded that the arthroscopic proximal pole scaphoidectomy and insertion of pyrocarbon spacer is an excellent procedure for the difficult and unsalvageable scaphoid nonunion.

Implant arthroplasty for unsalvageable scaphoid nonunion has a rich and storied history dating back to World War Two. Multiple generations and designs have been described. Although encouraging outcomes have been reported with complete scaphoid replacement with Swanson's titanium design, current preferred techniques include resection of the proximal pole and placement of a spacer. Current data suggest the pyrolytic carbon implant is preferred. These procedures have the advantage of being simpler than complex bone grafting techniques, requiring less rehabilitation and preserving options for salvage later.

References

1. Drac P, Manak P, Pieranova L. Distal scaphoid resection arthroplasty for scaphoid nonunion with radioscaphoid arthritis. Biomed Pap Med Fac Univ Palacky Olomouc Czech Repub. 2006;150(1):143–5.
2. Malerich MM, Clifford J, Eaton B, et al. Distal scaphoid resection arthroplasty for the treatment of degenerative arthritis secondary to scaphoid nonunion. J Hand Surg Am. 1999;24(6):1196–205.
3. Soejima O, Iida H, Hanamura T, et al. Resection of the distal pole of the scaphoid for scaphoid nonunion with radioscaphoid and intercarpal arthritis. J Hand Surg Am. 2003;28(4):591–656.
4. Ruch DS, Papadonikolakis A. Resection of the scaphoid distal pole for symptomatic scaphoid nonunion after failed previous surgical treatment. J Hand Surg Am. 2006;31(4):588–93.
5. Garcia-Elias M, Lluch AL, Farreres A, et al. Resection of the distal scaphoid for scaphotrapeziotrapezoid osteoarthritis. J Hand Surg Br. 1999;24(4):448–52.
6. Matsuki H, Horii E, Majima M, et al. Scaphoid nonunion and distal fragment resection: analysis with three-dimensional rigid body spring model. J Orthop Sci. 2009;14(2):144–9.
7. Beutel FK, Welk E, Martini AK. Long-term outcome of partial prosthesis management of proximal scaphoid pseudarthroses with a comparison of different follow-up protocols. Handchir Mikrochir Plast Chir Organ Deutschsprachigen Arbeitsgemeinschaft Handchir Organ Deutschsprachigen Arbeitsgemeinschaft Mikrochir Peripher Nerven Gefäße Organ Ver Dtsch Plast Chir. 1999;31(3):162–6; discussion 167–8.
8. Boeckstyns ME, Kjaer L, Busch P, et al. Soft tissue interposition arthroplasty for scaphoid nonunion. J Hand Surg Am. 1985;10(1):109–14.
9. Daruwalla ZJ, Davies K, Shafighian A, et al. An alternative treatment option for scaphoid nonunion advanced collapse (SNAC) and radioscaphoid osteoarthritis: early results of a prospective study on the pyrocarbon adaptive proximal scaphoid implant (APSI). Ann Acad Med Singapore. 2013;42(6):278–84.
10. Egloff DV, Varadi G, Narakas A, et al. Silastic implants of the scaphoid and lunate. A long-term clinical study with a mean follow-up of 13 years. J Hand Surg Br. 1993;18(6):687–92.
11. Gras M, Wahegaonkar AL, Mathoulin C. Treatment of avascular necrosis of the proximal pole of the scaphoid by arthroscopic resection and prosthetic semireplacement arthroplasty using the pyrocarbon adaptive proximal scaphoid implant (APSI): long-term functional outcomes. J Wrist Surg. 2012;1(2):159–64.
12. Haussman P. Long-term results after silicone prosthesis replacement of the proximal pole of the scaphoid bone in advanced scaphoid nonunion. J Hand Surg Br. 2002;27(5):417–23.

13. Leslie BM, O'Malley M, Thibodeau AA. A forty-three-year follow-up of a vitallium scaphoid arthroplasty. J Hand Surg Am. 1991;16(3):465–8.
14. Pequignot JP, Lussiez B, Allieu Y. A adaptive proximal scaphoid implant. Chir Main. 2000;19(5):276–85.
15. Spingardi O, Rossello MI. The total scaphoid titanium arthroplasty: a 15-year experience. Hand (N Y). 2011;6(2):179–84.
16. Swanson AB, de Groot SG, DeHeer DH, et al. Carpal bone titanium implant arthroplasty. 10 years' experience. Clin Orthop Relat Res. 1997;342:46–58.
17. Waugh RL, Reuling L. Ununited fractures of the carpal scaphoid: preliminary report on the use of vitallium replicas as replacements after excision. Am J Surg. 1945;67(2):184–200.
18. Legge RF. Vitallium prosthesis in the treatment of the carpal navicular fracture. West J Surg Obstet Gynecol. 1951;59(9):468–71.
19. Picaud A [Acrylic prosthesis in therapy of old pseudarthrosis of the carpal scaphoid]. Mem Acad Chir (Paris). 1953;79(8–9):200–3.
20. Agerholm JC, Lee ML. The acrylic scaphoid prosthesis in the treatment of the ununited carpal scaphoid fracture. Acta Orthop Scand. 1966;37(1):67–76.
21. Agner O. Treatment of non-united navicular fractures by total excision of the bone and the insertion of acrylic prostheses. Acta Orthop Scand. 1963;33:235–45.
22. Swanson AB. Silicone rubber implants for the replacement of the carpal scaphoid and lunate bones. Orthop Clin North Am. 1970;1(2):299–309.
23. Carter PR, Benton LJ, Dysert PA. Silicone rubber carpal implants: a study of the incidence of late osseous complications. J Hand Surg Am. 1986;11(5):639–44.
24. Kleinert JM, Stern PJ, Lister GD, et al. Complications of scaphoid silicone arthroplasty. J Bone Joint Surg Am. 1985;67(3):422–7.
25. Smith RJ, Atkinson RE, Jupiter JB. Silicone synovitis of the wrist. J Hand Surg Am. 1985;10(1):47–60.
26. Bentzon PG, Randlov-Madsen A. On fracture of the carpal scaphoid; a method for operative treatment of inveterate fractures. Acta Orthop Scand. 1945;16(1):30–9.
27. Qvick LI, Wilhelm KH. Tendon interposition arthroplasty after resection of necrotic carpal bone. Aust N Z J Surg. 1980;50(3):272–7.
28. Cook SD, Thomas KA, Kester MA. Wear characteristics of the canine acetabulum against different femoral prostheses. J Bone Joint Surg Br. 1989;71(2):189–97.
29. Grandis C, Berzero GF. Partial scaphoid pyrocarbon implant: personal series review. J Hand Surg Eur. 2007;32(Suppl. 1):95.

Chapter 22
Scaphoid Nonunion Advanced Collapse: Denervation

M. Haerle, T. Del Gaudio

Case Presentation

A 50-year-old right-hand dominant architect complained about increasing pain in his left wrist over the past couple of years. At first, the pain manifested only during dumbbell workouts, especially when the wrist was loaded in dorsiflexion. The patient described a condition of moderate rest pain (VAS 2-3). Under minor load sudden severe pain (VAS 8-9) appeared. His functional impairment consisted of a decrease in grip and pinch strength and a progressive limitation of range of motion in his left wrist. The current symptoms did not appear to be related to trauma, but the patient reported a sports accident 20 years before with wrist pain for several weeks at that time. No care was provided at that time.

Physical Assessment

On our clinical examination of the left wrist, we found normal skin and soft tissue. The assessed range of motion was decreased for palmar flexion/dorsiflexion (25/25°), as well as for radial/

M. Haerle (✉) · T. Del Gaudio
Clinic for Hand and Plastic Surgery, Orthopedic Clinic of Markgroeningen, Markgroeningen, Germany
e-mail: Max.Harle@okm.de

© Springer International Publishing Switzerland 2015
J. Yao (ed.), *Scaphoid Fractures and Nonunions,*
DOI 10.1007/978-3-319-18977-2_22

251

ulnar deviation (20/30°). Pain was produced in the radiocarpal joint during wrist motion, mostly when forcing dorsiflexion; less during radial deviation. The scaphoid-shift test was positive. Tenderness was elicited in the anatomic snuffbox. Neither pain nor tenderness was found in the scaphotrapezio-trapezoidal joint or in the thumb basal joint. A stable condition was found in the distal radioulnar joint (DRUJ), and TFCC stress tests were negative.

Diagnostic Studies

The radiographs (Figs. 22.1 and 22.2) reveal an unstable nonunion of the left scaphoid with dorsal intercalated segmental instability (DISI) deformity and a degenerative osteoarthritis (OA) between the scaphoid and the radial styloid process with concomitant marginal osteophytes. Overall, there is a decrease in carpal height with advanced OA between the head of the capitate and the lunate. Signs of OA are barely found in the lunate fossa.

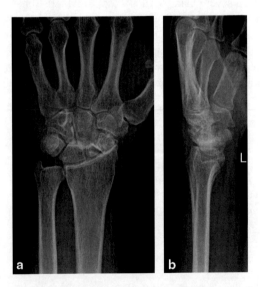

Fig. 22.1 Left wrist in two planes. (Published with kind permission of ©M. Haerle and T. Del Gaudio, 2015. All Rights Reserved)

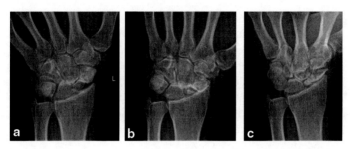

Fig. 22.2   Functional X-rays of the left wrist. (Published with kind permission of ©M. Haerle and T. Del Gaudio, 2015. All Rights Reserved)

Diagnosis

The conducted clinical and radiographical examinations (Figs. 22.1 and 22.2) were consistent with Stage III scaphoid nonunion advanced collapse (SNAC), mostly ascribable to a scaphoid fracture related to the previous sports accident.

Management Options and Management Chosen

Therapeutic decision-making in patients with SNAC wrist is based on a careful assessment of both the case history (taking account of patients age, profession, and dominant hand), as well as on the bone and cartilage status of the wrist, ascertained by radiographs and if indicated, by arthroscopy of the wrist, respectively. This allows a meaningful restriction of different conservative and surgical treatment approaches, such as nonunion repair, partial fusions of the carpus (e.g., four-corner fusion), proximal row carpectomy, wrist arthrodesis, radial styloidectomy, and wrist denervation[1].

In this specific case, we discussed in detail the clinical and radiological findings with the patient. Because of a radiological evident OA in the radiocarpal joint, no strategy of scaphoid repair was proposed. Proximal row carpectomy was contraindicated because of radiographic evidence of OA of the head of the capitate and in the midcarpal compartment. Since signs of OA between the lunate and the lunate fossa in the radiographs were scarce, we proposed to evaluate the intra-articular situation of the cartilage in the different joints by wrist arthroscopy. In case of intact cartilage layers between the lunate and lunate fossa, a four-corner fusion is alternatively proposed to wrist denervation as a salvage procedure. In case of cartilage damage in the lunate fossa, wrist denervation is more often chosen by patients before going to wrist arthrodesis.

Surgical Technique

Arthroscopy

The arthroscopy was performed with an upper-arm tourniquet. The hand was placed in stiff finger traps. 5 kg vertical traction was applied through a traction tower. First, the radiocarpal compartment was inspected through the 6R portal. Synovitis pervaded the radiocarpal compartment. The cartilage surface of the scaphoid and lunate fossa revealed grade IV chondromalacia, and the adjacent proximal articular surface of the lunate revealed grade II-III chondromalacia (Fig. 22.3).

Thereafter, the midcarpal compartment was inspected through the MCR portal which revealed grade II-III chondromalacia in the whole compartment, especially of the proximal pole of the capitate and the tip of the hamate (Fig. 22.4). It revealed OA with complete loss of cartilage due to the scaphoid nonunion.

Wrist Denervation in the Same Setting

Based on the arthroscopic findings and the assessed radiocarpal and midcarpal damages, we opted for complete wrist denervation as proposed by Wilhelm [2]. After removing the traction, the hand was placed on hand table for wrist denervation. A curved incision was performed on the dorsal distal forearm just proximal to the DRUJ (Figs. 22.5 and 22.6). Thereafter, the cutane-

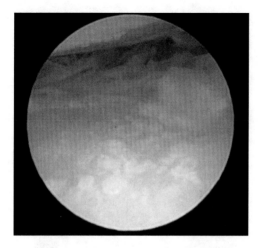

Fig. 22.3 Lunate fossa and counterfacing lunate. (Published with kind permission of ©M. Haerle and T. Del Gaudio, 2015. All Rights Reserved)

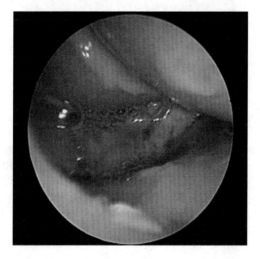

Fig. 22.4 Chondromalacia of capitate and hamate. (Published with kind permission of ©M. Haerle and T. Del Gaudio, 2015. All Rights Reserved)

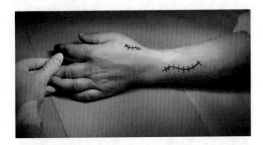

Fig. 22.5 Dorsal incision for denervation. (Published with kind permission of ©M. Haerle and T. Del Gaudio, 2015. All Rights Reserved)

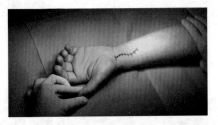

Fig. 22.6 Palmar incision for denervation. (Published with kind permission of ©M. Haerle and T. Del Gaudio, 2015. All Rights Reserved)

ous and subcutaneous layers are separated from the fascia layer. Perforating nerve branches were coagulated and transected. By doing so in proximal, distal, radial, and ulnar directions, the totality of the dorsal fascia was exposed like in a degloving injury. The fascia was incised in the area next to the muscle belly of the extensor pollicis longus. The muscle belly is retracted radially and the tissues lying on the interosseous membrane are exposed. A 2-cm segment of the posterior interosseous nerve (PIN) was coagulated and resected (Fig. 22.7). Next, a dorsoradial incision corresponding to the level of the trapeziometacarpal joint was made. The perforating branches originating from the superficial radial nerve and innervating the radial wrist capsule were coagulated and transected, protecting the cutaneous branches (Fig. 22.8). Another longitudinal incision was made just above the radial artery. The surrounding tissue was prepared in radio-

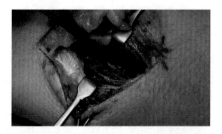

Fig. 22.7 Exposed posterior interosseus nerve. (Published with kind permission of ©M. Haerle and T. Del Gaudio, 2015. All Rights Reserved)

Fig. 22.8 Perforating branches of the superficial radial nerve. (Published with kind permission of ©M. Haerle and T. Del Gaudio, 2015. All Rights Reserved)

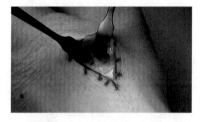

Fig. 22.9 Radial artery surrounded by periarterial tissue. (Published with kind permission of ©M. Haerle and T. Del Gaudio, 2015. All Rights Reserved)

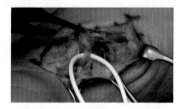

dorsal direction in order to create a communication with the previously prepared area on the dorsal side and to again interrupt the perforating branches of the superficial radial nerve. The radial artery was exposed using microsurgical technique and the periarterial tissue was coagulated and also resected (Fig. 22.9). Subsequently, the final volar incision was made. The palmar fascia was opened and the pronator quadratus muscle was lifted at the distal edge. Thereafter, the periosteum on the palmar aspect of the distal radius was removed under extensive coagulation. Branches of the anterior interosseous nerve (AIN) were intensively coagulated volar to the DRUJ. Following wound closure, postoperative immobilization was not necessary.

Clinical Course and Outcome

Four years following this procedure, the patient returned for a long-term follow-up. He reported to be free of complaints. The hand is used in everyday life, as well as in working life without any difficulties. In the clinical examination, the patient showed a range of motion of 25/30° for the palmarflexion/dorsiflexion and of 20/25° for radial/ulnar deviation. Upon loading the wrist, little pain was reported (VAS 1-2). DASH score was 5, compared to 70 preoperative.

Clinical Pearls/Pitfalls

- Denervation is indicated in painful wrist OA, preserving mobility.
- Wrist denervation represents a simple, low-risk surgical procedure. This procedure does not burn bridges and when compared to other wrist salvage procedures, it gives at least as good results.
- Preoperative testing gives results with little reproducibility and consequently low predictability. We therefore no longer perform these tests routinely.
- The PIN should be resected 1.5–2 cm proximal to the wrist, before it branches.
- The AIN may be dissected close to the distal rim of the pronator quadratus muscle and therefore just distal to the DRUJ.
- Resection of the AIN via a posterior approach, through the interosseous membrane following resection of the PIN, gives equivalent results. No patient to date has complained about the loss of function of the pronator quadratus.

- A meticulous dissection, coagulation, and interruption of as many perforating dorsal branches as possible by separating the superficial layers from the fascia on the complete dorsal aspect of the wrist helps the results of the denervation.

Literature Review and Discussion

Osteoarthritis (OA) of the wrist represents a relatively common painful condition with an overall prevalence of 1.7% in men and 1.0% in women [3]. If symptoms of OA persist or worsen despite of a conservative pain management (including NSAIDS, immobilization in a splint, or intra-articular injection of corticosteroids), surgical management for pain relief is taken into consideration. Apart from different salvage procedures described for patients with SNAC/SLAC wrist (e.g., partial midcarpal fusion and proximal row carpectomy), wrist denervation should be considered as an effective palliative surgical intervention, although it must be clear that the original pathology is not addressed. The best surgical indication is the patient with wrist pain in the presence of OA while there is still some preservation of wrist motion.

In fact, in terms of range of motion (ROM) none or minimal long-term postoperative impairment was reported after total wrist denervation only [4,5]. In contrast, partial carpal fusions and proximal row carpectomy are both associated with decreased ROM, ranging between 47–56% [6,7] and 43–63% [8,9] respectively, when compared to the contralateral wrist. Total wrist denervation has also been shown to provide a significant increase in grip strength. Rothe et al. showed in a collective of 46 patients (36 SNAC and 10 SLAC- wrists at stage II/III) an increase of 51% in grip strength after an average follow-up of 6.2 years [5].

In the literature, the reported overall pain relief after wrist denervation ranges between 56 and 85% [10,11]. In a study among 195 partial and total wrist denervations, 35% of patients achieved freedom from symptoms after a mean follow-up time of 4.1 years, and good results were achieved in 66% of cases [12]. Total wrist denervation, including AIN and PIN transection, seems to provide significantly higher pain reduction (76%) compared to PIN transection only (57%) [13, 14]. Interestingly, results of preoperative nerve blocking with local anaesthetics do not correlate with the postoperative degree of pain relief [13].

In summary, wrist denervation leads to significant pain reduction, preserving postoperative wrist mobility and improvement of grip strength. It therefore should be taken into account as a valid alternative to other salvage strategies such as (partial) fusions or PRC, when good wrist mobility is demonstrated preoperatively. Of course, denervation is not performed if any repair strategy can potentially delay or halt the progression of the disease. Also the interruption of afferent fibres can theoretically interrupt proprioceptive protective mechanisms, which are of relevance especially in younger patients, although this has not been shown in any clinical studies to date. In any case, these considerations may be neglected in cases of frank OA.

References

1. Shah CM, Stern PJ. Scapholunate advanced collapse (SLAC) and scaphoid nonunion advanced collapse (SNAC) wrist arthritis. Curr Rev Musculoskelet Med. 2013;6(1):9–17. doi: 10.1007/s12178-012-9149-4.
2. Wilhelm A. Die Gelenkdenervation und ihre anatomischen Grundlagen. Hefte Unfallheilkunde. 1966;86:1–109.
3. Haugen IK, Englund M, Aliabadi P, Niu J, Clancy M, Kvien TK, Felson DT. Prevalence, incidence and progression of hand osteoarthritis in the general population: the Framingham osteoarthritis study. Ann Rheum Dis. 2011;70(9):1581–6. doi: 10.1136/ard.2011.150078.
4. Schweizer A, von Känel O, Kammer E, Meuli-Simmen C. Long-term follow-up evaluation of denervation of the wrist. J Hand Surg Am. 2006;31(4):559–64.
5. Rothe M, Rudolf KD, Partecke BD. [Long-term results following denervation of the wrist in patients with stages II and III SLAC-/SNAC-wrist]. [Article in German] Handchir Mikrochir Plast Chir. 2006;38(4):261–6.
6. Wyrick JD, Stern PJ, Kiefhaber TR. Motion-preserving procedures in the treatment of scapholunate advanced collapse wrist: proximal row carpectomy versus four-corner arthrodesis. Hand Surg Am. 1995;20(6):965–70.

7. Dacho A, Grundel J, Harth A, Germann G, Sauerbier M. [Functional outcome after midcarpal arthrodesis in the treatment of advanced carpal collapse (SNAC-/SLAC-wrist)]. Handchir Mikrochir Plast Chir. 2005;37(2):119–25.

8. Baumeister S, Germann G, Dragu A, Tränkle M, Sauerbier M. [Functional results after proximal row carpectomy (PRC) in patients with SNAC-/SLAC-wrist stage II]. [Article in German] Handchir Mikrochir Plast Chir. 2005;37(2):106–12.

9. Jebson PJ, Hayes EP, Engber WD. Proximal row carpectomy: a minimum 10-year follow-up study. J Hand Surg Am. 2003;28(4):561–9.

10. Ekerot L, Holmberg J, Eiken O. Denervation of the wrist. Scand J Plast Reconstr Surg. 1983;17(2):155–7.

11. Geldmacher J, Legal HR, Brug E. Results of denervation of the wrist and wrist joint by Wilhelm's method. Hand. 1972;4(1):57–9.

12. Buck-Gramcko D. Denervation of the wrist joint. J Hand Surg Am. 1977;2(1):54–61.

13. Radu CA, Schachner M, Tränkle M, Germann G, Sauerbier M. [Functional results after wrist denervation]. [Article in German] Handchir Mikrochir Plast Chir. 2010;42(5):279–86. doi: 10.1055/s-0030-1249060.

14. Ishida O, Tsai TM, Atasoy E. Long-term results of denervation of the wrist joint for chronic wrist pain. J Hand Surg Br. 1993;18(1):76–80.

Chapter 23
Scaphoid Nonunion Advanced Collapse: Arthroscopic Debridement/ Radial Styloidectomy

Brandon P. Donnelly and A. Lee Osterman

Case Presentation

The patient was a 39-year-old right-hand-dominant male who presented with right wrist pain for several months. He was playing football and had a fall landing on his outstretched right hand. Previous to this, he had been diagnosed with a right scaphoid fracture 10 years ago also while playing football. This was initially treated with casting and subsequent bone stimulation. This initial fracture had gone on to nonunion and was subsequently treated with Russe bone grafting and K-wire fixation in which the patient was told the fracture healed. He noted that he had been asymptomatic for the previous 9 years after his wrist healed.

A. L. Osterman (✉)
The Philadelphia Hand Center, 700 S. Henderson Rd., Suite 200, King of Prussia, PA 19406 USA
e-mail: loster51@verizon.net

B. P. Donnelly
Pontchartrain Orthopedics and Sports Medicine, 3939 Houma Boulevard, Suite 21, Metairie, LA 70006, USA

© Springer International Publishing Switzerland 2015   263
J. Yao (ed.), *Scaphoid Fractures and Nonunions,*
DOI 10.1007/978-3-319-18977-2_23

Table 23.1 Grip strength in case of stage I scaphoid nonunion advanced collapse

	Right	Left
Flexion	75	90
Extension	70	85
Radial deviation	10	20
Ulnar deviation	25	40
Grip strength (lbs)	73	142

At our evaluation, the patient was able to localize the pain to the radial aspect of the wrist and described it as a sharp sticking pain. In addition, he noted worsening pain with wrist extension and push-off that limited both his work and leisure activities. He complained of weakness of his hand, especially when trying to hold or grip something heavy. He denied any numbness or tingling in his hand or fingers and has not had any treatment other than NSAIDs for pain.

Physical Assessment

On examination of the right wrist, there was mild dorsal radial swelling, boggy in nature, without any obvious deformity noted. Range of motion showed only mild limitations on the right compared to the left. Grip strength, however, was only 50 % of the unaffected arm (Table 23.1).

Palpation revealed tenderness over the anatomic snuffbox, dorsal scaphoid, and radial styloid. His pain was reproduced with radial deviation and dorsal radial motions of the wrist. The Watson shift maneuver produced pain without obvious clunk. There was negative lunotriquetral ballottement and TFCC stress testing. He had full composite digital motion and a normal neurovascular examination.

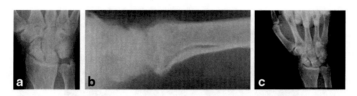

Fig. 23.1 Preoperative posteroanterior **a** and lateral **b** and power grip **c** radiographs consistent with SLAC stage 1. Note the extended position of the lunate in Fig 23.1b consistent with a DISI deformity. During grip, there is impaction of scaphoid on the arthritic radial facet of the radius. (Published with kind permission from © Brandon P. Donnelly and A. Lee Osterman, 2015. All Rights Reserved.)

Diagnostic Studies

Standard radiographs show a nonunited scaphoid waist fracture. Changes consistent with stage I SNAC wrist were present with beaking of the radial styloid and degenerative change and loss of joint space within the styloid–scaphoid articulation. The lateral radiograph revealed a classic dorsal intercalated segmental instability (DISI) pattern with a scapholunate angle of 85° (Fig. 23.1a, 23.1b). Radial styloid–scaphoid impingement was visualized with a clenched fist PA radiograph (Fig. 23.1c).

Diagnosis

Stage I Scaphoid Nonunion Advanced Collapse (SNAC) with radial styloid–scaphoid arthritis.

Management Options

We often find patients with early SNAC wrist to be relatively asymptomatic and as such may be treated with simple observation. Additional nonoperative measures include short-term immobilization as well as corticosteroid injections and other modalities.

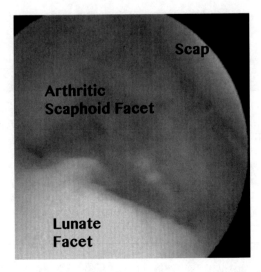

Fig. 23.2 Arthroscopic view of the radial styloid arthrosis from the 3–4 portal. The scaphoid is at 2 o'clock, and the lunate facet is at 7 o'clock. (Published with kind permission from © Brandon P. Donnelly and A. Lee Osterman, 2015. All Rights Reserved.)

Operative treatment includes radial styloidectomy, either open or arthroscopic. Denervation may also be an option. Bone grafting and open reduction of the scaphoid may also be performed with early SNAC wrists. In cases with more advanced radial scaphoid or scaphocapitate arthritis, a partial wrist fusion may be necessary.

Management Chosen

The patient underwent standard wrist arthroscopy, which showed a chronic scaphoid waist nonunion. Degenerative changes were noted about the distal aspect of the scaphoid and the radial styloid (Fig. 23.2). The remaining weight-bearing portion of the scaphoid and lunate facets of the radius did not show significant arthritic changes. The scaphocapitate and capitolunate joints were free of degenerative change as well.

In this case, with isolated radial styloid–scaphoid arthritis, an arthroscopic radial styloidectomy was performed. A standard wrist arthroscopic setup was used. The wrist was placed in 10 pounds of traction using finger traps and a traction tower. The customary 3–4 portal was employed for visualization, and a 1–2 portal was the working portal. Using the 2.7- or 2.3-mm arthroscope, a thorough diagnostic evaluation was done. Additional pathology may be addressed at this time prior to performing the styloidectomy, which may produce bleeding and debris that can impede visualization. In this case, no other concomitant pathology was noted. A small joint 3.5- or 2.9-mm burr was then used through the 1–2 portal to complete the resection with care taken to protect the radial extrinsic ligaments. Direct visualization and fluoroscopy was and should be used to ensure adequate amount of resection, approximately 3–4 mm. In addition, the diameter of the burr can be used as a reference to help guide resection.

After completion of the styloidectomy, the patient was placed in a short-arm volar splint for 7–10 days until initial postoperative follow-up. Gentle motion is begun at this visit, with limited activity for 6 weeks, followed by a gradual return to normal use. At 6 weeks postoperatively, the patient was released to increase his activities as tolerated and a strengthening program was begun.

Clinical Course and Outcome

The patient noted early improvement of his radially sided wrist pain. Pain relief was most notable with push-off and power grip. At 3-year follow-up, the patient was pain free. He had returned to his normal job as well as normal sporting activities. Range of motion had improved in all directions. There was also dramatic improvement of his grip strength (Table 23.2). X-rays showed a

Table 23.2 Grip strength after treatment

	Right	Left
Flexion	80	90
Extension	75	85
Radial deviation	15	20
Ulnar deviation	35	40
Grip strength (lbs)	135	130

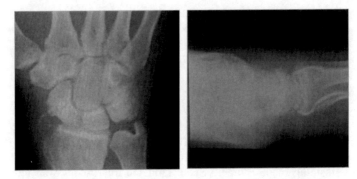

Fig. 23.3 Postoperative posteroanterior **a** and lateral **b** radiographs at 3-year follow-up. Note the level of resection. (Published with kind permission from © Brandon P. Donnelly and A. Lee Osterman, 2015. All Rights Reserved.)

persistent nonunion but a stable wrist with improvement in his DISI deformity (Figs. 23.3a, 23.3b).

Clinical Pearls/Pitfalls

- When performing any arthroscopic wrist procedure, a full diagnostic arthroscopy should be completed including both radiocarpal and midcarpal joints.
- Using a working 1–2 portal gives easier access to the radial styloid for excision; however, care must be taken when making the portal as not to injure the branches of the dorsal radial sensory nerve. This is done by incising only the skin and using a blunt hemostat to dissect down to and penetrate the capsule.
- When performing the styloidectomy, fluoroscopy should be used to assess the amount of resection. It is imperative that no more than 3–4 mm of styloid be removed as to not destabilize the wrist. The RSC and LRL ligaments should also be visualized and protected during excision.
- The dorsal branch of the radial artery is at risk.
- Radial styloidectomy is contraindicated in case with known radial carpal instability evidenced by ulnar translocation of the carpus, or in patients with incompetence of radial extrinsic ligaments.

Literature Review and Discussion

Radial styloidectomy was initially described by Barnard and Stubbins in 1948 in conjunction with fixation and bone grafting of scaphoid nonunion [1]. It has also been performed as an adjunct in the treatment of Kienböck's disease and late SLAC and SNAC wrist as there is potential for impingement of the carpus with the radial styloid after proximal row carpectomy, triscaphe and midcarpal athrodeses [2–4].

Anatomically, the radial styloid is volar to the midcoronal plane of the wrist and supports the scaphoid in extension and ulnar deviation. The styloid is also the origin of the radial extrinsic ligaments, which play a role of radiocarpal stability, most notably preventing ulnar translocation of the carpus. These volar extrinsic ligaments include the radioscaphocapitate (RSC) and long radial lunate (LRL) ligaments. The dorsal radial carpal ligament (DRC), also known as the radiolunotriquetral ligament, arises from the radial styloid as well. The RSC originates just 4 mm from the styloid process, and the LRL is located only 10 mm from the tip of the styloid[5–7].

A cadaveric study evaluating the incidence of wrist arthritis showed involvement to be most prevalent in the radial styloid and scaphoid articular surfaces [8]. Currently, the most common indication for radial styloidectomy is isolated arthritis at the radial styloid–scaphoid articulation. This occurs in the setting of radial styloid malunion, such as in cases of Chauffeur's fractures, or in early SNAC or SLAC wrist [9].

In both SNAC and SLAC wrist, there is alteration of the normal kinematics and force transmission across the radiocarpal joint. In SNAC, the free distal pole of the scaphoid moves independently of the proximal pole and adjoined lunate. This nonphysiologic motion decreases the contact area of the radioscaphoid articulation. This in turn leads to increased force over a smaller area and subsequent degenerative changes that begin along the radial styloid and distal scaphoid articulation [1]. Similar changes in kinematics from the carpal instability in SLAC wrists lead to the predictable pattern of degenerative changes associated with chronic scapholunate dissociation, which similarly arises first at the radial styloid–scaphoid joint.

In the early SNAC or SLAC wrist, with isolated arthritic change between the scaphoid and distal aspect of the radial styloid, a radial styloidectomy is indicated. After excision of the styloid, patients may enjoy significant pain relief from the unloading of that arthritic joint. Earlier techniques advocated open resection of the styloid; however, determining the extent of resection was always in question. Nakamura, in a cadaveric study, showed that excision of more than 4 mm of radial styloid sacrificed the important radial extrinsic ligaments, the RSC, and LRL and could lead to ultimate ulnar translocation of the carpus [10]. In some earlier work looking at open radial styloidectomy, it was determined that the short oblique osteotomy was the safest, and despite sacrificing the radial collateral ligament of the wrist, the more important RSC and LRL were preserved [7] (Fig. 23.4).

Arthroscopic radial styloidectomy is a good option in these cases of early wrist arthritis isolated to the radial styloid and scaphoid articulation. In addition to the evaluation of the area of concern, a more thorough investigation of the entire wrist joint may be performed and other pathology noted and addressed. A second benefit

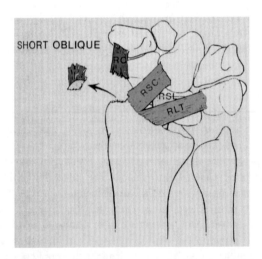

Fig. 23.4 Cartoon of the radial extrinsic ligaments at risk of iatrogenic injury during radial styloidectomy. An oblique styloidectomy was employed. (Published with kind permission from © Brandon P. Donnelly and A. Lee Osterman, 2015. All Rights Reserved.)

of arthroscopic resection is direct visualization of the styloid to be resected, as well as the important volar radial ligaments, which can then be protected from injury.

Complications of arthroscopic styloidectomy include incomplete and excessive resections. Also, destabilization of the wrist joint can occur with injury to the RSC and LRL ligaments, leading to ulnar translocation of the carpus [1, 10]. The dorsal radial sensory nerve is at risk with the 1–2 portal and should be avoided by incising only skin and using blunt dissection to approach the capsule and joint.

There is a paucity of literature evaluating isolated radial styloidectomy. However, there is some literature looking at combination of styloidectomy with other procedures. Stark and Herness achieved good relief of pain following open styloid excision performed in combination with ORIF of scaphoid nonunions [11, 12]. Kalainov et al. reported on seven patients with radioscaphoid arthritis, five of which underwent only arthroscopic radial styloidectomy. The remaining two had additional excision of the scaphoid. At an average of 2.5 years, two patients were pain free, and the other five complained of only mild, occasional wrist pain [13].

References

1. Barnard L, Stubbins SG. Styloidectomy of the radius in the surgical treatment of nonunion of the carpal navicular; a preliminary report. J Bone Joint Surg Am. 1948;30A(1):98–102. http://www.ncbi.nlm.nih.gov/pubmed/18921629. Accessed 13 Aug 2014.
2. Watson HK, Ryu J, DiBella A. An approach to Kienböck's disease: triscaphe arthrodesis. J Hand Surg Am. 1985;10(2):179–87. http://www.ncbi.nlm.nih.gov/pubmed/3980928. Accessed 19 Aug 2014.
3. Watson HK, Weinzweig J, Guidera PM, Zeppieri J, Ashmead D. One thousand intercarpal arthrodeses. J Hand Surg Br. 1999;24(3):307–15. doi:10.1054/jhsb.1999.0066.
4. Lin HH, Stern PJ. "Salvage" procedures in the treatment of Kienböck's disease. Proximal row carpectomy and total wrist arthrodesis. Hand Clin. 1993;9(3):521–6. http://www.ncbi.nlm.nih.gov/pubmed/8408264. Accessed 19 Aug 2014.
5. Blevens AD, Light TR, Jablonsky WS, et al. Radiocarpal articular contact characteristics with scaphoid instability. J Hand Surg Am. 1989;14(5):781–90. http://www.ncbi.nlm.nih.gov/pubmed/2794392. Accessed 19 Aug 2014.

6. Berger RA. The ligaments of the wrist. A current overview of anatomy with considerations of their potential functions. Hand Clin. 1997;13(1):63–82. http://www.ncbi.nlm.nih.gov/pubmed/9048184. Accessed 19 Aug 2014.

7. Siegel DB, Gelberman RH. Radial styloidectomy: An anatomical study with special reference to radiocarpal intracapsular ligamentous morphology. J Hand Surg Am. 1991;16(1):40–4. doi:10.1016/S0363-5023(10)80010-3.

8. Jeffries AO, Craigen MA, Stanley JK. Wear patterns of the articular cartilage and triangular fibrocartilaginous complex of the wrist: a cadaveric study. J Hand Surg Br. 1994;19(3):306–9. http://www.ncbi.nlm.nih.gov/pubmed/8077817. Accessed 19 Aug 2014.

9. Linscheid RL. Kinematic considerations of the wrist. Clin Orthop Relat Res. 1986;202:27–39. http://www.ncbi.nlm.nih.gov/pubmed/3955960. Accessed 19 Aug 2014.

10. Nakamura T, Cooney WP, Lui WH, et al. Radial styloidectomy: a biomechanical study on stability of the wrist joint. J Hand Surg Am. 2001;26(1):85–93. doi:10.1053/jhsu.2001.20963.

11. Stark HH, Rickard TA, Zemel NP, Ashworth CR. Treatment of ununited fractures of the scaphoid by iliac bone grafts and Kirschner-wire fixation. J Bone Joint Surg Am. 1988;70(7):982–91. http://www.ncbi.nlm.nih.gov/pubmed/3042793. Accessed 14 Aug 2014.

12. Herness D, Posner MA. Some aspects of bone grafting for non-union of the carpal navicular. Analysis of 41 cases. Acta Orthop Scand. 1977;48(4):373–8. http://www.ncbi.nlm.nih.gov/pubmed/335774. Accessed 14 Aug 2014.

13. Kalainov M, Cohen MS, Sweet S. Radial Styloidectomy. In: Geissler W, editor. Wrist Arthroscopy. 2005 edn. New York City: Springer; 2005, p. 134–8.

Chapter 24
Scaphoid Nonunion Advanced Collapse: Capitolunate Arthrodesis

R. Glenn Gaston and Matthew Wilson

Case Presentation

A 45-year-old right-hand-dominant male laborer was referred to the hand center with long-standing right wrist pain. The patient's past medical history was unremarkable, but he did admit to near-daily alcohol use and was a smoker. The patient initially injured his right wrist ~ 15 years prior to presentation while playing recreational volleyball. He was told he had a "hairline" fracture of the scaphoid and surgical intervention was recommended. The patient initially elected for nonoperative management. The pain in his right wrist continued to progress over the years to the point where presented with difficulty in grasping or reaching for objects. His pain was rated as an 8/10 on a visual analog scale, and he was unable to identify any alleviating factors.

R. G. Gaston (✉)
Department of Hand Surgery, OrthoCarolina Hand Center, 1915 Randolph Rd, Charlotte, NC 28207, USA
e-mail: Glenn.Gaston@orthocarolina.com; glenngaston@hotmail.com

M. Wilson
Carolinas Medical Center, Dept Orthopedic Surgery, Charlotte, NC, USA

© Springer International Publishing Switzerland 2015   273
J. Yao (ed.), *Scaphoid Fractures and Nonunions*,
DOI 10.1007/978-3-319-18977-2_24

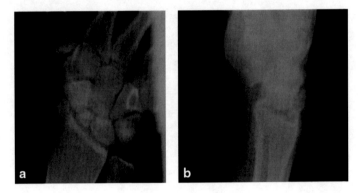

Fig. 24.1 a Postero-anterior (PA) image demonstrating stage 2 SNAC wrist.
b Lateral image of the same patient. DISI deformity noted as well. (Published
with kind permission of ©R. Glenn Gaston, 2015. All Rights Reserved). *PA*
Postero-anterior, *SNAC* scaphoid nonunion advanced collapse, *DISI* dorsal
intercalary segmental instability

Physical Assessment

Examination of the right wrist yielded significant tenderness to
palpation over the scaphoid in the anatomic snuffbox. There was
visible swelling noted as well over the dorsal–radial aspect of the
wrist. His range of motion in the sagittal plane was limited to 55°
of flexion and 30° of extension, but with relatively preserved pronosupination measuring 75° of supination and 90° pronation. He
was able to achieve pulp-to-palm contact, but was unable to make
a full composite fist. There was normal light touch sensation of the
fingers and brisk capillary refill.

Diagnostic Studies

The patient was presented to clinic with X-rays from his referring
provider (Fig. 24.1a, b). The radiographs demonstrated a proximal
third scaphoid nonunion with beaking of the radial styloid and
significant radioscaphoid and scaphocapitate arthrosis. His radiolunate and capitolunate joints appeared well preserved. A very small
separate facet on the lunate for the hamate was noted.

Diagnosis

Watson and colleagues described the evolution of arthritis in the wrist, but Vender and colleagues established the term scaphoid nonunion advanced collapse (SNAC) [1]. They described the stages as follows: stage I is characterized by arthrosis at the radial styloid–distal scaphoid articulation; stage II is characterized by involvement progressing to scaphocapitate arthrosis followed by stage III which is denoted by degenerative changes in the midcarpal joint—specifically, the capitolunate joint. Notably, the interface between the proximal pole of the fractured scaphoid and the radius is often spared. Based on the patient's history, physical examination, and diagnostic studies, the patient was diagnosed with stage II SNAC.

Management Options

- *Proximal row carpectomy (PRC)*: Proximal row carpectomy is a well-described method of managing scapholunate advanced collapse (SLAC) and SNAC wrist. Critical to its success is preservation of the articular surfaces of the lunate fossa and head of the capitate. Midcarpal arthrosis is a relative contraindication for this procedure. If PRC were selected, in that setting it would require either capsular interposition or an osteo-articular transfer system (OATS)-type procedure to be done concomitantly. PRC done for younger and higher demand patients is still controversial with advocates for and against its use in this patient cohort. Stern et al. have reported poorer outcomes in patients under 35 years of age but good results even in longer term studies of patients older than 35.
- *Midcarpal fusion*: There are many described techniques for scaphoid excision and midcarpal fusion including four-corner fusion (lunate, triquetrum, capitate, and hamate), three-corner fusion (fusing all except lunotriquetral (LT) joint), two-column fusion (sparing LT and capitohamate (CH) joints), and isolated capitolunate fusion. In principle, all are identical in that the scaphoid is removed and the midcarpal joint is stabilized with a

fusion. Proponents of the four-corner fusion cite a larger surface area for fusion as the main advantage. Studies have shown no difference in fusion rates, range of motion, and functional outcomes between the four-corner and isolated capitolunate techniques [2]. Advantages of an isolated capitolunate (CL) fusion include lower risk of subsequent pisotriquetral (PT) arthritis, less bone graft needs, less surgical time, and equal outcomes and union rates. In principle, the fewer number of joints necessary for fusion to be achieved assuming the other joints are free of degenerative change makes the most sense. Combined, these factors have led us to favor scaphoid excision and isolated capitolunate fusion with triquetral retention.

- *Malerich Arthroplasty*: This technique involves removal of the distal pole of the scaphoid (the portion distal to the nonunion). Long-term studies have shown very good results, and we do like this technique for some patients. The presence of midcarpal arthritis makes this technique less desirable, but it can work well in isolated stylo-scaphoid degeneration (SLAC I). It should be noted that preexisting DISI deformity often worsens after this procedure though it has not been correlated with worse outcomes in studies till date.

- *Denervation/Styloidectomy*: We use this procedure selectively in patients not wanting to undergo a larger procedure. Often, older or lower demand individuals do not want larger scale reconstructive procedures, and we will offer arthroscopic radial styloidectomy and anterior interosseous nerve (AIN)/posterior interosseous nerve (PIN) neurectomy.

- *Wrist arthrodesis*: For pancarpal arthritis, this is our procedure of choice. We also offer this if the patient has very poor pre-op read-only memory(ROM) (if less than roughly 30° arc of flexion/extension) as salvaging this small amount of motion and assuming the risk of possible additional future surgery does not seem worthwhile. Also patients with gout often present with apparent SLAC wrist that have had attenuation of the scapholunate (SL) over time and intraoperatively are found to have pancarpal arthritic change despite some radiographic joint preservation. These patients are counseled before surgery that midcarpal verses total wrist fusion may be needed depending on surgical findings.

- *Wrist Arthroplasty*: There are reports of successful management of wrist osteoarthritis using wrist arthroplasty. At our institution, we have abandoned wrist arthroplasty for osteoarthritis after poor outcomes were achieved, but still use it routinely for rheumatoid arthritis.

Management Chosen

Scaphoid excision and isolated capitolunate fusion with triquetral retention was chosen and is our procedure of choice for the majority of these patients. Critical factors in the decision include patient age/level of demand/comorbidities, preoperative ROM, and stage of disease. In lower demand patients, physiologically older patients, and those at higher risk of nonunion due to comorbidities, PRC is selected more often. Patients with pancarpal arthritis or very limited preoperative ROM are more often recommended total wrist fusion. Patients with very early degenerative changes (stage I), especially those who do not want to undergo a larger procedure, often undergo either Malerich arthroplasty +/− denervation (early SNAC) or arthroscopic radial styloidectomy with denervation (early SLAC). As mentioned above, we prefer isolated CL fusion with triquetral retention over four-corner fusion because of the lessened need for bone graft, lower risk of subsequent PT arthritis, shorter surgery time, and equivalent outcomes [2]. We now maintain the triquetrum as opposed to excising it, given the biomechanical data of increased load across the lunate associated with triquetral excision [3].

Clinical Course and Outcome

The patient underwent scaphoid excision and capitolunate arthrodesis approximately 1 month from the time of his initial evaluation. At his first postoperative visit, his surgical dressing was taken down and his sutures were removed. Active and passive range of motion of the wrist demonstrated smooth flexion, extension, ulnar, and

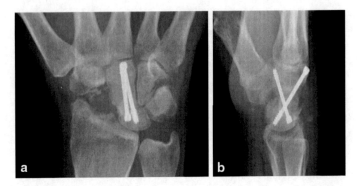

Fig. 24.2 a PA X-ray showing healing of the CL fusion without hardware migration. **b** Lateral X-ray showing healing of the CL fusion without hardware migration. (Published with kind permission of ©R. Glenn Gaston, 2015. All Rights Reserved)

radial deviation. He was placed into a short-arm cast and instructed to work on active range of motion exercises for the digits. He was counseled on smoking cessation. He returned to clinic at 6 weeks. At this visit, the patient admitted to performing repetitive heavy lifting and other vigorous activities with his operative extremity in spite of his ongoing restrictions. Radiographs were obtained and demonstrated intact hardware with a healing arthrodesis of the capitolunate joint (Fig. 24.2). The patient was placed into a removable splint, which he was instructed to use for all activities. A CT scan was ordered 3 months postoperatively to assess the arthrodesis site. The CT scan demonstrated intact hardware with bony bridging across the arthrodesis site between the capitate and lunate (Fig. 24.3). At the time of his final follow-up visit, the patient was no longer requiring narcotic pain medication, was able to perform all activities of daily living with minimal discomfort, and was anxious to return to work without restrictions. On examination, the patient's incision was well healed without signs of infection, he had full and supple range of motion of his digits, and his wrist range of motion measured 15° of extension, 45° of flexion, 80° of pronation, and 80° of supination. The patient was released to full duty at 4 months postoperatively.

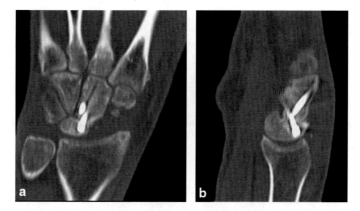

Fig. 24.3 a Coronal CT scan image showing bridging bone across the CL joint. **b** Sagittal CT scan image showing bridging bone across the CL joint. (Published with kind permission of ©R. Glenn Gaston, 2015. All Rights Reserved)

Clinical Pearls/Pitfalls

1. Reduce the lunate: Attaining colinearity of the lunate and capitate is critical and can be difficult at times. The DISI deformity can be challenging to reduce. Threaded K-wires into the lunate to use as joysticks followed by a single capitolunate pin is typically all that is needed. Also maximal passive wrist flexion, then driving a K-wire across the radiolunate joint with subsequent extension of the wrist and then advancing the wire across the midcarpal joint can work as well in difficult cases (Fig. 24.4).
2. Avoid hardware complications: K-wires alone for CL fusion have had an unacceptably high nonunion rate. Cannulated compression screws have a higher union rate but have been reported in multiple studies to back out and require repeat surgery for removal. When possible, retrograde screw placement is preferred so that the radiocarpal joint is not damaged with screw backout if this complication does arise (Fig. 24.5). Some patients have a very flat dorsal capitate head/neck morphology which makes retrograde screws very hard to place because of the difficult angle, and we do not prefer violating the 3rd carpometacarpal (CMC) as other authors have reported. Also getting two screws side by

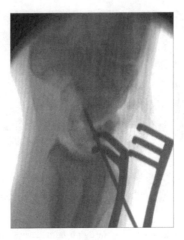

Fig. 24.4 Lateral X-ray demonstrating a K-wire having been advanced across the radiolunate and midcarpal joint to attain and maintain proper lunocapitate angle. (Published with kind permission of ©R. Glenn Gaston, 2015. All Rights Reserved)

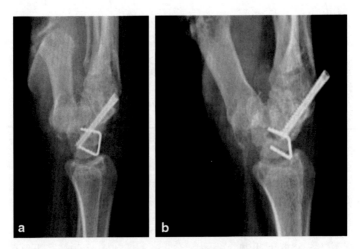

Fig. 24.5 **a** Lateral post-op X-ray with a staple and retrograde screw placed. **b** Lateral X-ray demonstrating back out of the retrograde screw. (Published with kind permission of ©Glenn Gaston, 2015. All Rights Reserved)

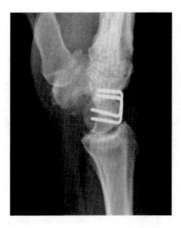

Fig. 24.6 Lateral X-ray showing well-seated staples in a small trough therefore not impinging on the dorsal rim of the distal radius. (Published with kind permission of ©R. Glenn Gaston, 2015. All Rights Reserved)

side can risk fracturing out the dorsal capitate cortex if the starting points are too close in more narrow capitate morphologies. In these cases, we will place antegrade screws (one or both) as needed. In patients who have a more deep, concave capitate head/neck, retrograde screws are easier to insert. We have more recently moved to nitinol memory staples for fixation. Making a small trough to bury the staple helps prevent dorsal impingement of the staple on the rim of the radius (Fig. 24.6).

3. Managing type 2 lunates: Type 1 lunates only articulate with the capitate and make this technique much easier. Some type 2 lunates have larger hamate facets making room for hardware in the capitate alone difficult. We have managed this with both excision of the proximal hamate and inclusion of the proximal hamate into the arthrodesis with no difference in outcome or complications noted till date (Fig. 24.7).

4. Bone graft: For isolated CL fusion, we have never required anything more than scaphoid cancellous bone for graft. The surfaces match well and do not require much grafting.

5. Joint preparation: We prefer to only use rongeurs and curettes for the joint preparation. We use no power in this part of the case as burrs often "polish" the surface and create unwanted heat even when copiously irrigated. Removing all subchondral bone

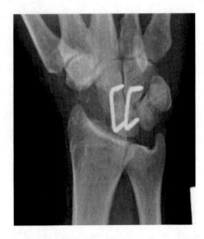

Fig. 24.7 PA wrist radiograph showing management of a type 2 lunate using one staple across the lunate–hamate joint. (Published with kind permission of ©R. Glenn Gaston, 2015. All Rights Reserved)

down to good cancellous bone is the key for attaining union. Typically, the lunate is more difficult to prepare given its concave shape and more often sclerotic bone.

Literature Review and Discussion

Four-corner fusion has been the traditional limited wrist fusion for SLAC and SNAC wrist based on the large surface area available for fusion and proven track record in published series. Interestingly, in Watson's original article on the management of SLAC wrist, three of his sixteen patients who underwent limited wrist fusions had a capitolunate fusion with results similar to the cohort having undergone four-corner fusion [4]. One of Watsons' first CL fusion patients was reported to have "rode 4753 miles on a bike with hand brakes" [5]. Isolated capitolunate fusion was first reported in 1966 for the management of Kienbocks [6] though early applications of this technique to the SLAC wrist were met with poor outcomes secondary to a high nonunion rate [7, 8]. The current four-corner fusion technique advocated by Watson arose from the desire to increase the surface area for fusion when compared to the isolated CL fusion. Refinements of the CL fusion technique (specifically changing fixation from K-wires to compression screws or compression staples) have greatly decreased the incidence of nonunion, and the technique offers the advantages of a lessened or even eliminated need for bone graft, and elimination of pisotriquetral arthritis as a complication [2, 9, 10]. While newer techniques continue to be reported, such as two-column fusions and other modifications to the traditional four-corner fusion, all require fusion of the triquetral–hamate joint. In our experience, this joint is rarely arthritic and fusing it has been shown to dramatically alter pisotriquetral mechanics as clinically evidenced by the late pisiform excision rates reported up to 33 % [2, 11]. This coupled with the success, and simplicity of an isolated capitolunate fusion with triquetral retention has reinforced our decision to continue this procedure as our procedure of choice for most SLAC and SNAC wrists.

References

1. Watson HK, Ryu J. Evolution of arthritis of the wrist. Clin Orthop Relat Res. 1986;202:57–67.
2. Gaston RG, Greenberg JA, Baltera RM, Mih A, Hastings H. Clinical outcomes of scaphoid and triquetral excision with capitolunate arthrodesis versus scaphoid excision and four-corner arthrodesis. J Hand Surg. 2009;34(8):1407–12.
3. Scobercea RG, Budoff JE, Hipp JA. Biomechanical effect of triquetral and scaphoid excision on simulated midcarpal arthrodesis in cadavers. J Hand Surg. 2009;34(3):381–6.
4. Watson HK, Ballet FL. The SLAC wrist: scapholunate advanced collapse pattern of degenerative arthritis. J Hand Surg. 1984;9(3):358–65.
5. Watson HK, Goodman ML, Johnson TR. Limited wrist arthrodesis. Part II: intercarpal and radiocarpal combinations. J Hand Surg. 1981;6(3):223–33.
6. Graner O, Lopes EI, Carvalho BC, Atlas S. Arthrodesis of the carpal bones in the treatment of Kienböck's disease, painful unfused fractures of the navicular and lunate bones with avascular necrosis and old fracture-dislocations of carpal bones. J Bone Joint Surg. 1966;48(4):767–74.
7. Kirschenbaum D, Schneider LH, Kirkpatrick WH, Adams DC, Cody RP. Scaphoid excision and capitolunate arthrodesis for radioscaphoid arthritis. J Hand Surg. 1993;18(5):780–5.

8. Krakauer J, Bishop A, Cooney W. Surgical treatment of scapholunate advanced collapse. J Hand Surg. 1994;19(5):751–9.

9. Calandruccio JH, Gelberman RH, Duncan SFM, Goldfarb CA, Pae R, Gramig W. Capitolunate arthrodesis with scaphoid and triquetrum excision. J Hand Surg. 2000;25(5):824–32.

10. Goubier JN, Teboul F. Capitolunate arthrodesis with compression screws. Tech Hand Up Extrem Surg. 2007;11(1):24–8.

11. Gaston RG, Lourie GM, Floyd WE, Swick M. Pisotriquetral dysfunction following limited and total wrist arthrodesis. J Hand Surg. 2007;32(9):1348–55.

Chapter 25
Scaphoid Nonunion Advanced Collapse: Scaphoid Excision and 4-Corner Arthrodesis

Nathan T. Morrell and Arnold-Peter C. Weiss

Case Presentation

A 45-year-old male CEO of a financial firm presented with a 3 year history of gradually worsening wrist pain. He recalled injuring his wrist in his 20's. A physician told him he had broken a "wrist bone" and he had worn a cast for 2 months. He had not had much pain until 3 years ago when he first noticed pain with exercise and weightlifting progressing to pain with most activities of daily living at present. He noticed that he has lost range of wrist motion and also noticed a "hard bump" on the dorsal-radial aspect of the wrist. He has tried a wrist splint, anti-inflammatory medicines and has had a corticosteroid injection into the wrist, all only providing short term relief of symptoms.

A. - P. C. Weiss (✉) · N. T. Morrell
University Orthopedics, Providence, RI 02905, USA

A. C. Weiss
Department of Orthopaedics, Alpert Medical School
of Brown University, Providence, RI, USA
e-mail: arnold-peter_weiss@brown.edu

© Springer International Publishing Switzerland 2015
J. Yao (ed.), *Scaphoid Fractures and Nonunions,*
DOI 10.1007/978-3-319-18977-2_25

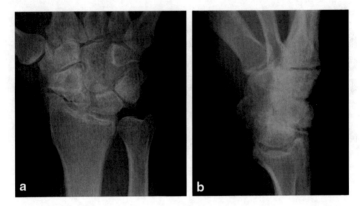

Fig. 25.1 Posteroanterior **a** and lateral **b** radiographs demonstrate an old scaphoid nonunion with findings of advanced collapse. (Published with kind permission of © Nathan T. Morrell and Arnold-Peter C. Weiss, 2015. All rights reserved)

Physical Assessment

On physical examination, there was swelling localized to the dorso-radial aspect of the wrist. There was tenderness to palpation about the scaphoid. Wrist range of motion was limited to extension of 30° and flexion of 35°; he had minimal radial and ulnar deviation of the wrist. There were no neurologic or vascular deficits. There was no erythema or overt signs of infection. Grip strength was about 30 % less than his uninjured wrist.

Diagnostic Studies

Posteroanterior and lateral radiographs were obtained demonstrating a scaphoid nonunion with atrophy of the proximal pole fragment, substantial radioscaphoid arthritis and erosion of the radioscaphoid joint contour. The radiolunate joint appeared intact and there was no significant erosion of the capitolunate joint articulation. Carpal height was collapsed on the lateral radiograph (Fig. 25.1a, b).

Diagnosis

Based on the history, physical exam, and radiographs, the diagnosis of scaphoid nonunion advanced collapse (SNAC), stage II was made. The development of degenerative changes following scaphoid nonunion progresses in a characteristic manner, much like in chronic scapholunate ligament insufficiency. Stage I SNAC involves the radial styloid-scaphoid articulation; Stage II involves the scaphocapitate interface, as well as progression of degeneration in the radioscaphoid articulation; and finally Stage III SNAC involves the capitolunate interface with progression of the previously involved joints. Generally, the proximal radioscaphoid and radiolunate articulations are preserved in true SNAC wrists [1]. Stage IV represents pan-carpal arthritis.

Management Options

Initial treatment for SNAC wrist should almost always be conservative. Activity modification, splinting, nonsteroidal anti-inflammatory medications, and intra-articular corticosteroid injections may be beneficial. Surgical intervention may be indicated when conservative treatment has failed.

Reasonable surgical treatments for advanced SNAC wrist include proximal row carpectomy, scaphoid excision with four-corner arthrodesis, total wrist arthrodesis, and total wrist arthroplasty, although the latter two options are usually reserved for Stage IV disease. For Stage II disease, either a proximal row carpectomy (PRC) or a scaphoid excision and four corner fusion are appropriate treatment options. In younger (less than 50 years of age) patients, we recommend a four corner fusion as the longevity of the radiolunate joint is quite predictable once a solid fusion occurs. The longevity of the capitate head articulation in younger patients following PRC is less predictable with subsequent arthritis a relatively more common finding. In older patients (more than 60 years of age), we generally recommend a proximal row carpectomy. In between 50 and 60 years of age, we favor four corner fusions in active individuals and proximal row carpectomies in the more sedentary.

Scaphoid excision with four-corner arthrodesis is contraindicated in the presence of radiolunate degenerative changes or radiolunate instability (e.g., ulnar carpal translocation due to radioscaphocapitate or long radiolunate ligament insufficiency), as well as in the presence of active infection.

Management Chosen

Scaphoid excision with four-corner arthrodesis, with use of a dorsal four corner fusion specific plate and autologous distal radius cancellous bone graft.

Clinical Course and Outcome

Following cast immobilization for 4 weeks and hand therapy for range of motion and strengthening for another 4 weeks, the patient returned to activities of daily living without restriction. At 3 months postoperative, the patient resumed golfing and tennis. Occasional aching in the wrist was noted for the first 3–4 months which ultimately resolved. Radiographs taken at 4 months demonstrated a solid four corner fusion and excellent plate recession (Fig. 25.4a, b) Follow-up examination at 6 months will generally demonstrate range of motion (ROM) of 35° wrist extension and 30° of wrist flexion. In general, wrist flexion lags wrist extension. By 1 year postoperative, average wrist ROM = extension 45° and flexion 35°. Average grip strength at 1 year is 75 % of the contralateral hand. VAS pain scores at 1.5 out of 10 at 6 months and 0.9 out of 10 at 1 year.

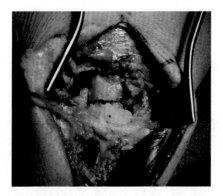

Fig. 25.2 All four joints being fused need to have complete debridement down to good and bleeding cancellous bone at each joint carefully removing all hard subchondral bone and cartilage. (Published with kind permission of © Nathan T. Morrell and Arnold-Peter C. Weiss, 2015. All Rights Reserved)

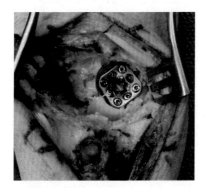

Fig. 25.3 The plate should be recessed below the level of the fusion mass with careful placement of all the screws (lag=*gold* and locking=*blue*) into each of the four bones being fused. (Published with kind permission of © Nathan T. Morrell and Arnold-Peter C. Weiss, 2015. All Rights Reserved)

Clinical Pearls/Pitfalls

While a number of different fixation techniques have been described (e.g., K-wires, screws, staples, various plates, etc.), a good functional result following four-corner arthrodesis is likely more due to

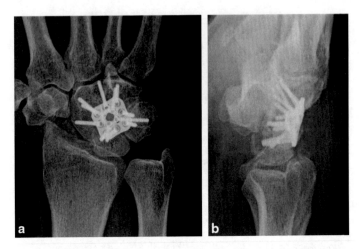

Fig. 25.4 Final posteroanterior **a** and lateral, **b** radiographs should demonstrate excellent consolidation of the fusion mass, carpal alignment and plate recession. (Published with kind permission of © Nathan T. Morrell and Arnold-Peter C. Weiss, 2015. All Rights Reserved)

technical factors than specific implant or fixation technique chosen [2]. We believe that an adequate amount of quality bone graft is critical; we recommend distal radius autogenous cancellous bone. We caution against the use of the morselized scaphoid as bone graft as this poor quality bone may have contributed to previously reported elevated nonunion rates [2].

Additionally, adequate preparation of the articular interfaces is critical. All cartilage from at least the dorsal two thirds of each intercarpal joint must be removed to bleeding, subchondral bone (Fig. 25.2). After reaming or drilling, any debris must be removed from the intercarpal interstices so as to allow for adequate contact and compression of the fusion surfaces.

When using a dorsal plate for fixation, the plate must be appropriately sized and positioned in the appropriate location. All screws must have good purchase and we prefer plates with locking screws for added postoperative stability (Fig. 25.3). Care must be taken to avoid too long of screws in the triquetrum which may penetrate the pisotriquetral joint possibly causing pisotriquetral pain. All four corners of the carpal bones must meet; the triquetrum tends to migrate ulnarly and may need provisional fixation. To avoid dorsal impingement of the plate, the preoperative DISI deformity, if present, must be corrected. Provisional Kirschner wire (K-wire) fixation may be helpful [2, 3]. Lastly, careful attention to reaming is paramount. The lunate is often harder bone than the hamate or capitate and may cause the reamer to tilt distally; as such, we recommend keeping the pressure on the lunate while reaming.

Literature Review and Discussion

The primary goal of treatment for SNAC wrists is pain relief while maintaining some wrist range of motion and improving strength. Scaphoid excision with four-corner arthrodesis has proven a reliable treatment for advanced SNAC [4].

A systematic review of outcomes indicates that good pain relief can be expected with scaphoid excision and four-corner arthrodesis with approximately 90 % of patients being satisfied with the procedure [4]. Postoperative grip strength averages approximately 75 % of the uninvolved contralateral side [4].

Regarding wrist range of motion, in vitro analysis of wrists suggested that approximately 36 % of wrist flexion-extension would be lost with a four corner fusion due to the loss of mid-carpal motion[5]. In practice, approximately 40–55 % or wrist flexion-extension is typically lost when compared to the uninvolved, contralateral wrist [1, 2]

The overall complication rate with four-corner arthrodesis is approximately 13 % [3]. The most common complication is nonunion. The historical nonunion rate is around 8 %, however with recent techniques and particular attention to detail, this rate has approached zero [2]. Other complications include: dorsal radiocarpal impingement; superficial or deep infection; reflex sympathetic dystrophy; injury to the superficial branch of the radial nerve; and others [3].

References

1. Enna M, Hoepfner P, Weiss AP. Scaphoid excision with four-corner fusion. Hand Clin. 2005;21:531–8.
2. Merrell GA, McDermott EM, Weiss AP. Four-corner arthrodesis using a circular plate and distal radius bone grafting: a consecutive case series. J Hand Surg Am. 2008;33:635–42.
3. Shin AY. Four-corner arthrodesis. J Am Soc Surg Hand. 2001;1:93–111.
4. Mulford JS, Ceulemans LJ, Nam D, Axelrod TS. Proximal row carpectomy vs four corner fusion for scapholunate (Slac) or scaphoid nonunion advanced collapse (Snac) wrists: a systematic review of outcomes. J Hand Surg Eur Vol. 2009;34:256–63.
5. Gellman H, Kauffman D, Lenihan M, Botte MJ, Sarmiento A. An in vitro analysis of wrist motion: the effect of limited intercarpal arthrodesis and the contributions of the radiocarpal and midcarpal joints. J Hand Surg Am. 1988;13:378–83.

Suggested Reading

Weiss KE, Rodner CM: Osteoarthritis of the Wrist. J Hand Surg Am. 2007;32:725–46.

Chapter 26
Proximal Row Carpectomy for Scaphoid Nonunion Advanced Collapse Wrist

Olukemi Fajolu and Charles Day

Case Presentation

A 40-year-old right-hand-dominant male who fell onto his out-stretched hand 9 months prior to presentation presented with persistent right wrist pain. He had been out of work secondary to his injury. He described his pain as a 3/10 at baseline, and an 8/10 with activity. He had been wearing a removable wrist splint that did help control some of his symptoms. He denied any numbness, tingling, or weakness. He endorsed a smoking history of half a pack per day of cigarettes. He denied the use of illicit drugs or significant alcohol use.

C. Day (✉) · O. Fajolu
Department of Orthopaedic Surgery, Beth Israel Deaconess
Medical Center, Harvard Medical School, 330 Brookline Ave,
Stoneman 10, Boston, MA, USA
e-mail: cday1@bidmc.harvard.edu

© Springer International Publishing Switzerland 2015
J. Yao (ed.), *Scaphoid Fractures and Nonunions,*
DOI 10.1007/978-3-319-18977-2_26

Physical Assessment

Examination of the right hand and wrist revealed significant swelling and tenderness over the anatomic snuffbox. He had limited wrist range of motion with 10° of extension, 15° of flexion, 10° of radial deviation, and 15° of ulnar deviation. Motor and sensory examinations were intact in all nerve distributions.

Diagnostic Studies

On the initial evaluation with the patient, X-rays were obtained of the right wrist demonstrating a scaphoid waist nonunion with sclerosis of the proximal pole (Fig. 26.1). The patient was sent for an MRI of his wrist demonstrating a scaphoid nonunion with signal changes concerning for avascular necrosis of the proximal pole (Fig. 26.2). There was associated medial scaphoid, radial styloid, radial carpal, and radioscaphoid arthritis. The MRI revealed intact

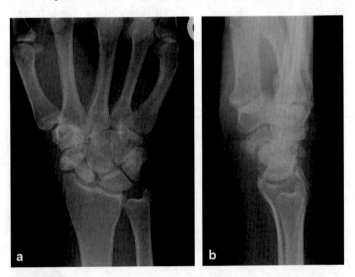

Fig. 26.1 a and **b** posteroanterior and lateral preoperative radiographs. There is evidence of radioscaphoid arthrosis. (Published with kind permission of © Olukemi Fajolu and Charles Day, 2015. All Rights Reserved)

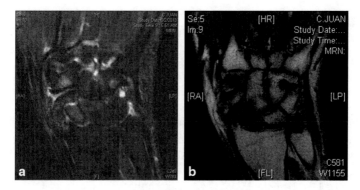

Fig. 26.2 a Coronal *T2*-weighted and **b** coronal *T1*-weighted MRI scans revealing decreased signal within the proximal pole of the scaphoid concerning for avascular necrosis. (Published with kind permission of © Olukemi Fajolu and Charles Day, 2015. All Rights Reserved)

cartilage at the head of the capitate and very mild capitolunate arthritic changes. The position of the lunate also revealed a DISI deformity (Fig. 26.3).

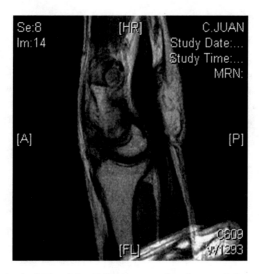

Fig. 26.3 Sagittal *T1*-weighted MRI scan revealing the extended posture of the lunate consistent with a DISI deformity. (Published with kind permission of © Olukemi Fajolu and Charles Day, 2015. All Rights Reserved)

Diagnosis

The patient was diagnosed with scaphoid nonunion advanced collapse (SNAC) given findings on both X-ray and MRI. A SNAC wrist pattern of arthritis develops from a scaphoid nonunion that goes untreated. Given the blood supply of the scaphoid, which is predominantly retrograde, proximal pole fractures are more at risk for developing a nonunion. Scaphoid fractures that go untreated and result in nonunions are at risk for developing a DISI (dorsal intercalated segment instability) deformity as well as a SNAC wrist. [1, 2] In stage I of SNAC, the arthritis is localized to the distal scaphoid and the radial styloid. In stage II, this progresses to the radioscaphoid joint. Stage III involves the midcarpal joint, specifically the scaphocapitate and capitolunate joints. Stage IV involves pancarpal arthritis. As a general rule, the proximal lunate is often spared, as is the lunate fossa. This patient was diagnosed with SNAC stage II.

Management Options

In general, treatment for SNAC wrist is largely determined based on the stage of the condition. For stage I SNAC wrist, treatment options include excision of distal scaphoid and radial styloidectomy with possible fixation of scaphoid nonunion with bone graft. A distal scaphoid resection, also known as the Malerich procedure [3], is a possible procedure for this early stage of SNAC because it allows the patient to mobilize quickly after surgery, does not require any bony healing, and allows for subsequent surgeries, should the patient's arthritis progress. For stage II SNAC wrist, options include salvage procedures such as a PRC, 4-corner arthrodesis, and total wrist arthrodesis. For stage III SNAC wrist, options include 4-corner fusion as well as total wrist arthrodesis and total wrist arthroplasty.

Management Chosen

Proximal row carpectomy (PRC) was described in 1944 by Stamm [4]. Among the salvage procedures, PRCs and 4-corner fusions are the most motion-preserving operations. When comparing a PRC to a 4-corner fusion, however, findings in the literature have been varied. While there are some studies that that have shown more motion preservation after a PRC. There are others that suggest they have similar ROM outcomes [5–7]. In a proximal row carpectomy, the scaphoid, lunate, and triquetrum are excised, and the capitate comes to articulate with the lunate fossa of the distal radius. The lunate fossa of the distal radius and the lunate more closely match in terms of their radii of curvature. The capitate, however, has a slightly different radius of curvature, and thus, a PRC leaves a translational component to the new articulation[8].

One of the contraindications of a PRC is significant cartilage wear in the head of the capitate. It is also ill-advised in patients with inflammatory arthritis or collagen disorders. Given the absence of cartilage wear on the capitate in our patient, the decision was made to proceed with a PRC. In addition, the patient's smoking history presents potential difficulty for him to heal from an arthrodesis procedure. We discussed the risks, benefits, and alternatives of the procedure, and the patient underwent a PRC for his SNAC wrist without event.

Surgical Technique

In a proximal row carpectomy, these are typically approached from either a transverse or longitudinal dorsal incision. Our preference is to use a longitudinal incision made over the dorsum of the wrist ulnar to Lister's tubercle. The extensor retinaculum is then incised over the 3rd dorsal extensor compartment. The capsulotomy may be performed in various ways. It is our preference to perform the capsulotomy with an inverted-T, reflecting the capsule off the carpus. A posterior interosseous neurectomy is typically performed to help decrease postoperative wrist pain. If significant synovitis

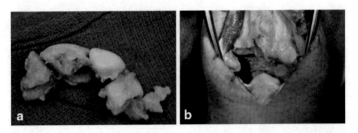

Fig. 26.4 a and **b** Compete excision of the proximal carpal row. (Published with kind permission of © Olukemi Fajolu and Charles Day, 2015. All Rights Reserved)

exists upon inspection of the joint, a synovectomy is typically performed, which was the case in our patient.

The head of the capitate as well as the lunate fossa should be inspected once the midcarpal and radiocarpal joints are exposed, to ensure there is no cartilage wear on these surfaces. We prefer to provide longitudinal traction in order to inspect these surfaces prior to proceeding with a PRC. If there is significant arthritis at these surfaces, an alternative procedure should be considered. As a general rule, we consent patients for all possible procedures, in the event that the arthritis is more extensive than initially thought, based on the preoperative MRI images. The lunate, triquetrum, scaphoid nonunion site, and all associated osteophytes should be removed in their entirety (Fig. 26.4). It is our typical fashion to do this with a combination of sharp dissection with a Beaver blade as well as a rongeur. Fluoroscopy is used to confirm the proper identification of the carpal bones prior to excision. It is also used to confirm complete excision of the carpal bones at the end of the procedure (Fig. 26.5). Of note, it is important when performing a PRC that the radioscaphocapitate (RSC) ligament, which runs from the distal–volar lip of the radius to the capitate, be preserved, as it functions to keep the capitate reduced in the lunate fossa, preventing ulnar translation of the carpus. Particular attention to this detail is most important when performing a radial styloidectomy, which is often done if there is carpal impingement on the radial styloid.

Once the carpal bones are excised, one needs to ensure that there is adequate reduction of the capitate in the lunate fossa. The capsular tissue and the extensor retinaculum are then closed using

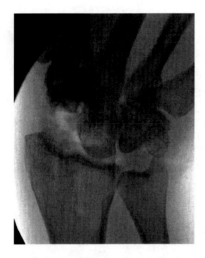

Fig. 26.5 Fluoroscopic image following the proximal row carpectomy. The capitate head is concentrically reduced within the lunate facet. (Published with kind permission of © Olukemi Fajolu and Charles Day, 2015. All Rights Reserved)

interrupted 3−0 Vicryl sutures. Skin and subcutaneous tissues are closed in layers. We prefer to place patients in a short-arm dorsal splint and have the wrist positioned extended and in an ulnarly deviated position. X-rays are then checked under fluoroscopy after the splint is placed, and the wrist is verified to be in a well-reduced position

Clinical Course and Outcome

Postoperatively, the patient's pain was well controlled. He was sent to occupational therapy 10 days postoperatively to work on digit ROM. He maintained reduction of his capitate on the lunate fossa (Fig. 26.6). Dedicated wrist range of motion therapy began at 4 weeks postoperatively, with the intent to advance to strengthening as tolerated. At 3 months postoperative, the patient was returned to full activity without restriction which is the routine follow-up of this procedure. Typical range of motion following this procedure is

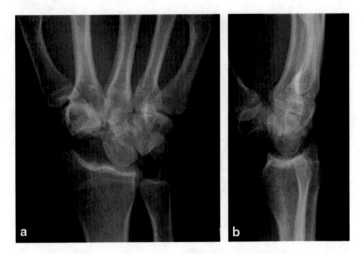

Fig. 26.6 a and **b** Final follow-up radiographs revealing maintenance of the position of the capitate within the lunate facet. (Published with kind permission of © Olukemi Fajolu and Charles Day, 2015. All Rights Reserved)

within 50–70% of the contralateral side, which is what the patient demonstrated at the final follow-up.

Clinical Pearls/Pitfalls

- In the setting of a scaphoid nonunion, an MRI may help determine the quality of the blood supply to the proximal pole.
- When evaluating a patient with a SNAC wrist, it is valuable to obtain advanced diagnostic studies, such as an MRI or CT scan to further evaluate for any associated arthritis in the carpus and the condition of the cartilage for any wear patterns, as this will help you determine treatment options.
- When the cartilage on the proximal pole of the capitate is well preserved, a PRC is a reliable treatment option.
- It is important to not violate the radioscaphocapitate ligament (RSC) during this procedure and to ensure proper reduction of the capitate on the lunate fossa.

- Verify that the scaphoid, lunate, and triquetrum are completely excised.
- If performing a radial styloidectomy at the same time or in isolation for early stages of SNAC, this should be limited to 5 mm, so not to disrupt the RSC ligament.

Literature Review and Discussion

Patients with SNAC wrist often present with wrist pain localized to the radial aspect of the wrist. Oftentimes, there is swelling and tenderness at the radioscaphoid joint. The patient may or may not remember an inciting event. Typically, there is a decrease in wrist motion, especially radial deviation and extension, stemming from the DISI deformity. A decrease in grip strength is also a common complaint and clinical finding. When approaching a patient with scaphoid nonunion advanced collapse, there are many treatment options available to the physician. These include wrist denervation, radial styloidectomy, excision of the distal pole of the scaphoid, proximal row carpectomy, scaphoid excision with 4-corner arthrodesis, and total wrist arthrodesis. PRC preserves some motion for the patient, in comparison with a total wrist arthrodesis. In addition, although it has been shown that some motion is lost after a PRC, resulting in a flexion–extension arc of 84° and radioulnar deviation arc of 43°, this was not significant enough to prevent patients from activities of daily living. [9, 10] In a systematic review looking at follow-up over 10 or more years, PRC has been shown to exhibit long-term durability.[11] In addition, it has been shown that although radiocapitate arthritis may develop radiographically over time, clinically this may be asymptomatic.

References

1. Mack GR, et al. The natural history of scaphoid non-union. J Bone Joint Surg Inc. 1984;66:504–9.
2. Ruby LK, et al. The natural history of scaphoid non-union. J Bone Joint Surg Inc. 1985;67-A:428–32.

3. Gelberman R. The wrist: master techniques in orthopaedic surgery. 3rd ed. Philadelphias: LWW; 2010.

4. Stamm T. Excision of the proximal row of the carpus. Proc R Soc Med. 1944;38:74–5.

5. Wyrick JD, Stern PJ, Kiefhaber TR. Motion-preserving procedures in the treatment of scapholunate advanced collapse wrist: proximal row carpectomy versus four-corner arthrodesis. J Hand Surg Am. 1995;20:965–70.

6. Cohen MS, Kozin SH. Degenerative arthritis of the wrist: proximal row carpectomy versus scaphoid excision and four-corner arthrodesis. J Hand Surg Am. 2001;26:94–104.

7. Dacho AK, Baumeister S, Germann G, Sauerbier M. Comparison of proximal row carpectomy and midcarpal arthrodesis for the treatment of scaphoid nonunion advanced collapse (SNAC-wrist) and scapholunate advanced collapse (SLAC-wrist) in stage II. J Plast Reconstr Aesthet Surg. 2008;61:1210–8.

8. Imbriglia JE, Broudy AS, Hagberg WC, McKernan D. Proximal row carpectomy: clinical evaluation. J Hand Surg. 1990;15:426–30.

9. Palmer AK, Werner FW, Murphy D, Glisson R. Functional wrist motion: a biomechanical study. J Hand Surg Am. 1985;10:39–46.

10. Ryu JY, Cooney WP 3rd, Askew LJ, An KN, Chao EY. Functional ranges of motion of the wrist joint. J Hand Surg Am. 1991;16:409–19

11. Chim H, Moran SL. Long term outcomes of PRC: a systematic review of the literature. J Wrist Surg. 2012;1(2):141–8.

Suggested Readings

Dacho AK, et al. Comparison of proximal row carpectomy and midcarpal arthrodesis for the treatment of scaphoid nonunion advanced collapse (SNAC-wrist) and scapholunate advanced collapse (SLAC-wrist) in stage II. J Plast Reconstr Aes Surg 2008;61:1210e1218.

Daruwalla ZJ, et al. An alternative treatment option for scaphoid nonunion advanced collapse (SNAC) and radioscaphoid osteoarthritis: early results of a prospective study on the pyrocarbon adaptive proximal scaphoid implant (APSI). Ann Acad Med. 2013;42(6):278-84

Stamm T. Excision of the proximal row of the carpus. Proc R Soc Med. 1944;38:74–5.

Erratum to: Scaphoid Nonunion Advanced Collapse: Capitolunate Arthrodesis

Matthew Wilson Chapter 24: *Scaphoid Nonunion Advanced Collapse: Capitolunate Arthrodesis,* which appears in Scaphoid Fractures and Nonunions, J J. Yao (ed.), Scaphoid Fractures and Nonunions, DOI 10.1007/978-3-319-18977-2_24, contained an error in the author name in both printed and electronic versions. The error has been corrected and is reflected in both print and electronic versions.

The online version of the original chapter can be found under:
http://dx.doi.org/10.1007/10.1007/978-3-319-18977-2_24

Matthew Wilson
Carolinas Medical Center, Dept Orthopedic Surgery, Charlotte, NC, USA

© Springer International Publishing Switzerland 2015   E1
J. Yao (ed.), *Scaphoid Fractures and Nonunions,*
DOI 10.1007/978-3-319-18977-2_27

Erratum to:
Unsalvageable Scaphoid Nonunion: Implant Arthroplasty

Alessio Pedrazzini Chapter 21: *Unsalvageable Scaphoid Nonunion: Implant Arthroplasty,* which appears in Scaphoid Fractures and Nonunions, J J. Yao (ed.), Scaphoid Fractures and Nonunions, DOI 10.1007/978-3-319-18977-2_21, had wrong order of authors and photo credits in both printed and electronic versions. The error has been corrected and is reflected in both print and electronic versions.

The correct order of authors and photo credits are given below:

Marco Rizzo, Alessio Pedrazzini and Maurizio Corradi

The updated original online version for this chapter can be found at
http://dx.doi.org/10.1007/978-3-319-18977-2_21

© Springer International Publishing Switzerland 2018   E3
J. Yao (ed.), *Scaphoid Fractures and Nonunions,*
DOI 10.1007/978-3-319-18977-2_28

Erratum to:
Scaphoid Fractures and Nonunions

Alessio Pedrazzini FM/List of contributors: J. J. Yao (ed.), Scaphoid Fractures and Nonunions, DOI 10.1007/978-3-319-18977-2, missed to include an author in both printed and electronic versions. The error has been corrected and is reflected in both print and electronic versions.

The authors and affiliation detail is given below:

Alessio Pedrazzini, MD Department of Orthopaedic Surgery and Traumatology, Oglio Po Hospital, Cremona, Italy

---

The updated original online version for this chapter can be found at
http://dx.doi.org/10.1007/978-3-319-18977-2

© Springer International Publishing Switzerland 2018   E5
J. Yao (ed.), *Scaphoid Fractures and Nonunions,*
DOI 10.1007/978-3-319-18977-2_29

Index

© Springer International Publishing Switzerland 2015
J. Yao (ed.), *Scaphoid Fractures and Nonunions*,
DOI 10.1007/978-3-319-18977-2

Printed in the United States
By Bookmasters